Sex Guide For Couples

How To Give Each Other Mind-Blowing Sexual Experiences

(3-in-1 Book)

Book 1: Sex Guide For Men: Orgasm Manual - Shoot Her To The Moon And Back

Book 2: Sex Guide for Women: F*ck Him Beyond His Wildest Dreams - Mentally, Physically & Emotionally

Book 3: Sex Guide For Women: The Roadmap From Sleepy Housewife to Energetic Woman Full of Sexual Desire

By: Ashley Williams and More Sex More Fun Book Club

Introduction Book 1

Ah, the orgasm! That sexual ideal and destination which pretty much all men seem to reach, but which seems to remain elusive for plenty of women. It has, in turn, frustrated, excited and confounded but always fascinated the human mind. It has thrown up controversies, shown shocking new facts and made us look at female sexuality very differently over the ages.

But academic interest isn't what is going to help us achieve that much-longed for state of ecstacy. More importantly, it isn't going to get our partner there. So, do you find yourself wondering whether your lover is satisfied in bed? Perhaps you feel that you aren't doing enough to make your sexual life appealing to her. Perhaps you feel that you could do more. Have you wondered whether she faked her orgasm the last time you had sex?

Questions like these about an activity as intimate and closely related to our self-esteem as sex can cause several confidence-killing thoughts. That is where this book comes in. We will examine the female orgasm and all its types in great detail. But this isn't just a technical study. Oh no, that wouldn't help our cause at all. This book is about how to ensure that you and your partner enjoy making love and both of you get maximum pleasure from the act.

We will look at different techniques, old and new. We will examine mental states and how they affect a woman's ability to orgasm. We will learn the effects of communication and lack thereof in terms of a satisfying sexual encounter or a sex life. Most of all, we will look at how you and your partner can have a happier, healthier and more rewarding sexual life.

You don't have to wait to finish the book to start using the advice I give you here. You can start incorporating the changes I recommend as soon as you read them. The point here is to give you a guide that helps you understand your partner's sexual wants, use that understanding to improve your sex life and feel much more satisfied by it than you may feel at the moment.

Thank you for purchasing this book. I hope you have a pleasant time reading (and following) it.

Chapter 1: The History Of The Female Orgasm

Before we get to how you can pleasure your partner into sexual oblivion, you must understand the way the female orgasm has been perceived throughout the centuries. You may not be aware of it, but the way the big O has been seen with regards to women may have colored your thinking too. While it is a history of repression, it is not solely so. The female orgasm has also gone through periods where great interest was shown. However, only now is it even remotely close to being understood.

Contrary to popular belief, during the medieval times, the female orgasm was considered absolutely necessary to procreation. Medieval scientists believed that a woman needed to orgasm in order to be able to have a child. From the 13th century onwards, the scientific theory held that for the sexual act to be fruitful, a woman must climax during the act. The notion was based on the belief that a woman's sexual organs were exactly like a man's, but they were inverted. This meant that women ejaculated just as men did during sex, the only difference being that they ejaculated inwards.

In the 1800s, sexual tension in women was diagnosed as hysteria. It was also known as wandering womb. The condition was thought to be specific to women and hence was also often called female hysteria. It was believed that the condition would drive a woman completely insane unless it was treated. The mode of treatment? Clitoral stimulation.

Women were supposed to masturbate in the privacy of their homes. Those women who were unable to climax received genital massages from physicians. Eventually, these physicians went on to invent the vibrator to make their job easier.

The 1940s brought with them Alfred Kinsey's explosive surveys about people's sexual behavior. Suddenly, the female orgasm wasn't a mysterious and perhaps even mythical phenomenon at all. The Kinsey Report showed that 40 percent of the women who were surveyed masturbated and had achieved their first orgasm that way. Other phenomena such as 'wet dreams,' multiple orgasms and the age at which women may lose the ability to orgasm were also discussed in the Report. While certain aspects of the Report have been debunked, it cannot be denied that the Kinsey Report was instrumental in busting a lot of sexual myths, especially as they related to women.

In the 1960s, now that the female orgasm was an established fact, plenty of studies and theories abounded about the necessity of the female orgasm. Various scientists theorized about why women orgasmed. Desmond Morris, in his book, *The Naked Ape*, theorized that the reason the female orgasm developed was so that women could select good mates and fathers based on qualities other than aggression and size, such as intelligence, care, imagination and patience. He also erroneously suggested that the female orgasm was meant to make the woman feel exhausted at the end of sex and keep her horizontal so that the sperm wouldn't leak out.

Other scientists believed that monogamy was not the goal or the reason for the female orgasm – in fact, it was quite the opposite. According to them, it was a way for women to bond with multiple sexual partners. Some others have speculated that the muscular contractions in the vagina during orgasm help conception by sucking up sperm. Others point out that if a woman achieves orgasm during sex, it is more likely that she will indulge in sex again, thus increasing the chances of conception.

Today, while the purpose of the female orgasm is still not clear, its benefits are definitely out there. It has been proved that orgasms in women improve the mood (naturally!), regulate the menstrual cycle, boost the immune system and the white blood cell levels, improve the functioning of the brain and work as great pain relievers.

So read on and find out how you can ensure that your partner enjoys all these benefits while both of you enjoy a stimulating sex life.

Chapter 2: The Ins And Outs Of The Female Orgasm

So, now that we're beginning, the first thing to know is what the female orgasm is all about. The NHS describes the female orgasm as "an intense, pleasurable release of sexual tension. It is accompanied by contractions of the genital muscles. A woman may be able to experience more than one orgasm shortly after the first if she continues to be stimulated."

So far so good. That sounds simple enough, doesn't it? But as you can tell from the previous chapter the female orgasm has been covered in so much myth and has been the subject of so much repression and misinformation that, today, 25% of women aren't even sure that they have achieved climax — either during sex or while masturbating. Quite a few women are sure that they cannot orgasm and a significant number state that they can only experience orgasm during masturbation and not during sexual intercourse.

All these statistics can be pretty daunting for their sexual partners. Therefore, the first thing to do is arm yourself with information. The first step to ensuring that your partner achieves the same satisfaction that you do during sex is to understand all the factors that govern the female orgasm. This is because unlike a man who is able to achieve orgasm only through physical stimulation, a woman's orgasm is affected by a combination of physical and mental factors. Let us take a look at what some of these factors are.

1. Physiological Factors

There are various physiological factors that can contribute to a woman's failure to climax. If you want to ensure that your partner achieves an orgasm during sex, you must be aware of what these factors are.

a) Age

Several studies conducted over the past few decades have found that the incidence of anorgasmia or the inability to orgasm is more prevalent among older women. While the reasons for this aren't well known, it is speculated that this happens because of the hormonal changes that happen with age such as a decrease in the level of estrogen and progesterone because of menopause. It is believed that the changes in the hormonal levels affect a woman's ability to achieve orgasm.

Certain psychological factors may also affect a woman's ability to climax in a sexual encounter as she ages. We will look at these factors in detail a little later.

b) Testosterone

Studies conducted on women and their hormonal levels have linked low levels of testosterone to a decreased ability to be aroused sexually and achieve orgasm. Couple this with the fact that about 70 million women around the world take the oral contraceptive pill which also reduces the testosterone levels in the female body, and it is not surprising that many doctors advise their female patients of the unofficial side effect of the pill – namely, a reduced sex drive and even an inability to achieve orgasm.

c) Estrogen

As mentioned earlier, menopause causes the levels of estrogen in the blood to go down. These lowered levels of the hormone have been linked to changes in sensations in the genitals and the blood flow to and from the genital area. In addition, decreased levels of estrogen also affect lubrication in the vagina and a woman's moods – both of which can explain a loss of interest in sex and an inability to achieve orgasm in menopausal and post-menopausal women.

d) Medical Conditions

Medical conditions can also affect a woman's ability to climax during sex. These conditions can cause more difficulty in achieving an orgasm, reduced frequency of orgasms and a change in how orgasms feel. These conditions include but are not limited to rectal disease, cancer, spinal cord injury, depression, anxiety and other such psychological disorders. Even hysterectomies have been known to adversely affect women's ability to orgasm.

e) Medications

Just as the medical conditions listed above can adversely affect a woman's ability to orgasm during intercourse, so too can the medicines required to treat those conditions. For example, women taking mood altering medicines such as anti-depressants used to treat depression, often complain about an inability to climax during sex or even a decreased sex drive. As mentioned above, the oral contraceptive pill has also been linked to a decreased ability to orgasm in women. There are, however, scientists who postulate that the pill actually benefits a woman's sex drive and her ability to climax. So far, both sides have produced inconclusive evidence to support their theories.

f)   Physical stimulation

Yup, this one is true lads. Studies have shown that women are much more likely to achieve climax when there is an adequate amount of foreplay involved. Exactly how much foreplay and for how long is different from woman to woman. We will discuss sexual techniques and positions that will maximize her pleasure, later on in the book.

In addition to foreplay, a whopping 95% of women have reported that they were much more likely to orgasm if clitoral stimulation rather than vaginal stimulation was utilized (only 26% in favor of vaginal stimulation).

2. Psychological factors

Apart from the physiological factors listed above, there are a number of psychological factors that can also affect women's ability to orgasm. These factors can arise from upbringing, social taboos, cultural conditioning, parental upbringing, sexual trauma and various other factors. Let's take a look at some of the prominent factors below.

a)   Body Issues

It is a fact that most women are unhappy with their bodies in some way or the other. This unhappiness and self-consciousness can intrude during sex and interrupt the build up to a climax. Thoughts can range from disparaging thoughts about one's body (I'm so fat, my breasts are too large/small, I'm too thin) to feelings of shame associated with the genital region (My vagina is too large/too small, I'm not clean so avoid oral sex, I'm too dry). Negative attitudes towards bodily functions that have been ingrained during toilet training tend to persist throughout one's life. This means that a lot of women see their bodies and specifically their genitals as 'dirty'. As such, they feel much more self-conscious during sex and are unable to enjoy the act enough to climax.

b)   Negative Attitudes Towards Sex

Growing up, many women acquire distorted views of sex. They get these views from society and from their families. Sex is viewed as bad or immoral. Attitudes towards nudity, sex play and even masturbation are severely negative and shameful and don't just affect women, but to a great extent, men as well. It's not surprising then that certain sexual acts are viewed as acceptable whereas others are 'kinky' or worse yet 'dirty' or taboo. Rigorous enforcement of religious belief systems too implies that sex is blasé or sinful, and we should strive to overcome it. All this conditioning results in women who believe that it is sinful, wrong and bad for them to seek out and enjoy sex. Not just that, but they believe that they deserve negative consequences and even punishment for daring to do so.

c) Mother-Daughter Bonds and Guilt About Breaking Them

This factor is not so well-known. For most young girls, their mothers are the ones they observe and imitate. As such, they are supremely uncomfortable with doing something that is different from what their role models do. This becomes even more apparent when it comes to a subject such as sex. If a mother is sexually repressed, her daughter will generally find it very difficult to go beyond her mother's boundaries when it comes to sexual fulfillment. The fear and guilt get transferred to other women with the result that most women do not want to stand out as sexually mature individuals.

d) Fear of Arousing Repressed Sadness

When women are in a sexual situation that is also emotionally intimate, they can experience sadness related to some childhood emotional pain. This becomes more acute for women who have experienced rejection or mistreatment early on in life. Such negative experiences are an absolute contrast to the feeling of being not only loved but also pleasured and fulfilled sexually. As such, women can experience very painful emotional responses while making love. If they try to hold these feelings back, they become cut off and detached from the sexual experience.

e)   Fear of vulnerability

While women are as capable of initiating and enjoying casual sexual encounters, when they start becoming more involved in a relationship they find that the love and positive acknowledgement can disturb their equilibrium psychologically speaking. These emotions can actually breach their defenses and leave them feeling acutely vulnerable. It brings to the fore that their happiness is dependent upon someone else. As such, they realize that they are wide open to emotional hurt and pain. If they have been hurt before, both men and women are very leery of courting such pain again by making themselves vulnerable. Thus, they hold themselves back during the sexual act and, in women, that can lead to an inability to climax.

f)   Abuse and Trauma

It has been estimated that one in every four women has been through inappropriate sexual contact either with strangers or with a relative or family members before she turned 18. As such, they can find themselves sub-consciously linking any sexual experience to their abuser, especially when the abuser is a relative, friend or family member – someone they thought they could trust. In such cases, sex becomes linked to feelings of guilt, revulsion and pain both physical and emotional and therefore, becomes unacceptable to a woman's mind. Unfortunately, such memories can be triggered through a position, things said during sex or even a certain look.

Whew! That's quite a lot, isn't it? The list of factors itself is daunting. Add into this the fact that most women take anywhere between 15 to 40 minutes to climax, and it is a wonder that women ever have an orgasm at all. But that is where you men come in. For the sexual experience to be truly enjoyable, it is essential that both parties enjoy what goes on in the bedroom (or the kitchen, dining room, shower, etc.). As such, we are now going to discuss techniques and positions that will not only help your partner achieve orgasm but also make sure that both of you enjoy the journey thoroughly.

Chapter 3: Types Of Female Orgasms

Yes, gentlemen, you heard right – there are types; and not just one or two, but four types. So for our first lesson in how to make her come, we are going to discuss the different types of orgasms a woman can have and how you can increase her chances to have that orgasm (or those orgasms; whatever, we're not picky).

Clitoral Orgasm

Ah, the clitoris! The confluence of eight thousand nerve endings! For most women, this bundle of nerves is what needs just the right touch to send them tumbling head first into a fantastic orgasm. Having said that, don't head straight for this little bundle. Stimulate other parts of her vagina by caressing and massaging them before you hone in on this little baby.

Techniques – You can make big circles with your fingers that touch upon the clitoral hood, the shaft and the labia. You can do this during foreplay. You can also do this if you're in the spoon position during intercourse. If you are performing oral sex on her, try lying perpendicular to her and thus approach her clitoris indirectly.

Increase her chances – Try using a fingertip vibrator. Encourage her to tell you what setting, speed, pressure and intensity she prefers. Also, try to experiment a bit and take note of her non-verbal cues.

Vaginal Orgasm

It has finally been established. The G-spot exists! This is good news for you lads because 30% of women say that they can come just from having this particular spot stimulated during penetrative sex. Locate, stimulate and enjoy!

Techniques – Of course, the first thing to do is to locate this famous spot. Explore the front wall of her vagina with your finger until you reach a part that feels spongy and rippled in texture. When you touch her there, you will probably see an immediate reaction (a good one). During intercourse, try making sure that you target your thrusting there. You can try lying on your sides facing each other. Intertwine your legs comfortably. Align your genitals and make sure that your penis rubs against the front wall of her vagina. The position ensures deeper thrusts that are more stimulating for the G-spot.

Increase her chances – Her chances of achieving a vaginal orgasm increases the longer the intercourse lasts. Try switching positions often during intercourse. This has a double advantage – it prevents you from coming too soon and helps her experience different and new sensations which can contribute to a vaginal orgasm. Try a warming lubricant for some extra help.

Blended Orgasm

So, as the name suggests, this one mixes the clitoral and the vaginal orgasms. Oh, mama! This one can be a really powerful and explosive finale. In fact, experts say that this is *the most* powerful one. It is estimated that this is twice as intense and strong as either of the other two. She will love you for this one.

Techniques – Girl on top – trust me on this one. There is a reason this one is so popular. It's perfect for this double finish. You can also have her sitting on your lap facing away from you. This way she controls the thrusting while you stimulate the clitoris. If you're doing the missionary, inch your body up so that your hips are aligned. Have her tilt her pelvis upward so that the base of your penis is on the clitoris but the rest of you is inside her. You're not thrusting up and down in this position. Instead, you're grinding against her pelvic bone.

Increase her chances – It's easier for a woman to have a blended orgasm if she becomes very aroused before actual intercourse. Foreplay is king here. You want to do lots of touching, kissing, massaging and licking all over. If you find that the feeling is waning a bit during intercourse, do the heavy petting again.

Multiple Orgasms

The first thing to understand here is what multiple orgasms really are. These are orgasms that happen one right after another. Orgasms that happen at different times during the same session aren't multiple orgasms (although they're still awesome). If your woman can stand being stimulated continuously after the first orgasm (and the second and the third and the fourth and so on), it is possible for her to have multiple orgasms.

Techniques – Start with foreplay. Use your fingers or mouth or a vibrator to get her to her first clitoral climax. Don't stop there, though. Immediately after she comes, you need to continue stimulating her clitoris. For the first 30 seconds do this slowly and then you can resume your normal pace to build her up to a climactic repeat performance. Basically, you're manipulating her level of arousal by easing off a bit when she is more sensitive and then building up the arousal again. From here you can begin intercourse. This can lead to multiple vaginal or even blended orgasms. Remember to use the same technique – slow down, speed up. Keep the stimulation going on and keep the arousal high.

Increase her chances – If she complains about feeling too sensitive, you can use a buffer. Stroke her over a buffer such as a pair of soft silk panties or a silk camisole. You can shift to her breasts and nipples for some time. These areas are quite sensitive, and you can push her to another orgasm simply by stimulating these areas.

Well, there you have it – four basic types of orgasms that women can have and how you can ensure that they have them. Don't think that you are required to master one or the other. The idea here is to explore and find what works for both you and her (especially her!). I hope you find this instructive (and fun – don't forget the fun!).

Chapter 4: Make Her Come

Finally, the chapter you've all been waiting for. In this one, we're going to look at how you can utilize each and every minute of your sexy time with her to ensure she is well taken care of and truly satisfied. Research at the Kinsey Institute shows that on average women take about ten to twenty minutes to climax. We're going to discuss some techniques that'll help you make sure she's still experiencing the aftermath of explosive orgasms well after your 15-minute quickie is over. Not only will it make you a sex god, but research also shows that a woman who has more orgasms will demand more sexy times with you (naturally!).

There is no rule that says you can't cheat a bit – and anyway, it isn't cheating if you don't touch. Subconscious foreplay is fair play. Meet up with her on a day when she has a yoga class, or take her out to a funny movie or a standup comedy show. Have some drinks at your place (or her place – whatever you've decided). Research shows that women are more aroused after they drink a glass or two of red wine. Set the mood and let's begin.

Kiss, Kiss, Kiss

Spend at least three minutes on kissing her thoroughly. Did you know that kissing actually reduces levels of cortisol, also known as the stress hormone, in your body? The more you kiss, the less stressed you are and the easier and faster it is for both of you to get turned on. Tilting your head to the right makes you seem more caring and makes her feel a connection with you. This, in turn, increases oxytocin in her system which encourages her to trust you and thus eventually come faster. Don't spend your time thinking about all this, though. Just enjoy the kiss!

There's More to Kissing than Just the Mouth

In a study of about fifty thousand women, 96 percent said that a kiss on the neck was the perfect way to warm up. Too much isn't good, though – the neck can become desensitized if you only focus there. Kiss her mouth and occasionally slide down to her neck.

At this point, you need to become coordinated. Every time you move down to kiss her neck, remove an item of clothing (hers definitely, yours maybe). Not only does this save you some time, but it also helps you deal with any body-confidence issues that she might have. Remember what we said earlier about how a woman can let her body issues interfere with her ability to enjoy her time with you? Well, this is the perfect way for you to ensure that you show *and* tell her that you love her body. As you remove her clothing, be sure to run your fingertips all over her body, around every curve and dimple she has to subconsciously reassure her mind you appreciate every inch of her body. Add in compliments as you remove each item of clothing. She will feel less self-conscious with each expression of your admiration and approval. Soon, you'll have the tigress you want in your bed (or her bed; again, not picky).

Tease Her Before You Please Her

Building the anticipation is super important. You've probably got most of her clothes off by now. Don't remove her underwear just yet. Yes, I know – it's tempting to head straight in. But patience brings rewards. Tease her by acting as though you have all the time in the world (which you do; this isn't a 100-meter dash). Build up the anticipation both in her and in yourself. Then remove her underwear. It's probably a good idea to use some scented lube at this point as it will excite her and sensitize her at the same time. Remember what we discussed earlier about clitoral orgasms. This is when you want to move your fingers in slow circles around and just inside her vagina.

Oral is Vital

Yes, boys, it is! Research shows that 80 percent of women say that it is the most reliable way for them to achieve the big O. Here's something called the Kivin Method that should get her there in a jiffy. Use one hand to pull up her clitoral hood. Lick the base of the hood, just above the clitoris, from side to side. In the meantime, put one finger of the other hand on the area just below her vaginal opening. You'll know that your finger is in the right place when you feel her pre-orgasmic contractions.

Entrance Exam

While foreplay is a crucial factor in her orgasm, it isn't the only one. Now that you have stimulated her to her first orgasm, intercourse is the next step since the length of the intercourse can determine the consistency of her orgasms. A study in the Journal of Sexual Medicine states that on an average she will climax about seven minutes after penetration. Therefore, now is the time to get started.

Worried about positions? Recall what we discussed about coital alignment technique. To recap, start in the missionary position. Then align your groins in such a way that the base of your penis rests on her clitoris. You want to grind against her pelvic bone, so try a backward and forward movement rather than a thrusting one. This not only massages her clitoris but also gives pulsating and slow sensations that are controlled by you.

You can also try the technique we discussed for the blended orgasm in the previous chapter by spooning her and using your hand or a toy to stimulate her clitoris while thrusting against her G-spot from behind.

Keep it Up

Oh yeah, don't change anything at this point. She should be going wild by now. You don't need anything new to get to the finishing point. You're doing it so just keep on doing it. Keep the speed and pressure the same and once the screaming, clawing climax is over, catch your breath because she's going to want more very soon.

Chapter 5: Positions That Will Work For Her Every Time

So now that we've covered the sex guide to make sure that her experiences with you leave her wanting more (and more and…), we can mix things up a bit. The same old, same old can get exactly that – old. You need to change things up from time to time, not just for her but for you too. At this point, I have to tell you a girl secret (that may not be a secret at all). Most women fake their orgasms – a lot. We know you want to please us, and we don't want to disappoint you. So we fake our orgasm or we just let you assume that we had one. But you don't have to settle for fake when you can blow her mind by giving her the real thing. Here are some positions you can try that will make her explode (in a good way) every time.

1. **Missionary**

Yes, that's right gentleman. The good old missionary is the one that works best for us. We get the most pleasure out of this old-fashioned position. It's close, it's intimate, it makes us feel cared for because your weight is on us and you surround us. You can make it even better for us by entering at the perfect angle. Don't come straight in. Instead, try a more diagonal approach. It achieves friction for the clitoris which is the best way to make a woman achieve orgasm.

2. **Reverse Cowgirl**

In this position, you are either in a sitting position or lying down. She straddles you backwards, meaning, she faces your feet instead of your head. This position allows you easy access to her clitoris and still gives her control over the thrusts. Not only will this get her a clitoral orgasm, but you can also even give her a blended one.

3. Doggy Style

This position is not just great for the man; it is also brilliant for the woman. It gives her a good amount of control. She can determine what angle is best for her and adjust her range of motion accordingly. You can stimulate her G-spot and her clitoris. Use your hand or a toy such as a small bullet vibrator. Don't just leave it up to the toy, though. Your hand is very important because remember, it's all about touch.

4. Girl on Top

This position is again a favorite because it allows her control of her own orgasm. This is basically the reverse of reverse cowgirl, so she's straddling you and facing your head. Encourage her to move in a backwards and forward motion instead of an up and down one – more stimulation for her clitoris. Don't just lie there, though. Join in by moving her hips. It gives more of an in sync feeling and makes for better communication – you know what she wants, and she knows what you want. Both of you work towards it together.

5. Spooning

In case she doesn't enjoy deep penetration (it can happen), try spooning. The efficacy of this technique can be seen in the fact that I've already mentioned it twice, and I'm talking about it again. It's fairly relaxed, so if you're into a lazy weekend morning play session, this position is perfect. The stimulation happens in the front wall of the vagina – yes that's right, the G-spot. At the same time, you can go for a blended orgasm by stimulating her clitoris.

6. Crisscross

This one is another great one if you want to focus on clitoral stimulation. Both of you need to lie down. You should be on your side, while she is on her back. Her legs are draped over your middle, kind of like a giant X. Either one of you can reach down and stimulate her clitoris since you're not squeezed against each other.

7. The Pillow Technique

It has been found by various sex experts and researchers that a woman finds sex more pleasurable when a pillow or a blanket is added into the mix because it makes for a new and different angle of entry. You can use the pillow in the missionary position by putting it under her bottom to raise her pelvis. This can help you stimulate her G-spot upon penetration. Not every angle will be comfortable for her so find out what works for her and use that.

8. Coital Alignment Technique

You knew I was going to bring this baby back! Just like the spooning, this is a great position to ensure mutual enjoyment and fulfillment. Some have even called it the 'greatest sexual position in the world'. It was created by psychotherapist Edward Eichel and involves you lying in missionary not resting your weight on your arms. You need to move so that the base of your penis is in direct contact with her clitoris. Remember to lock her legs around your thighs. Use a rocking rather than a thrusting motion. This position works out great not just because of the clitoral stimulation but also because it is physically the closest position.

9. Ankles Up

Moving her legs around can help because sometimes being on top of her or flat on her will not give you the penetration both of you need. In this position, you put her ankles up on your shoulders. This allows for a much deeper penetration and ensures you hit her G-spot with every thrust. You can also do this by bending her knees or putting her feet flat on your chest.

10. Kneeling

This is another woman on top position. You sit in an armchair or on the bed, and she kneels on the chair or bed, straddling you. She controls not just the penetration but also when both of you will climax by deciding the speed, grind and thrust to suit her own (and your) pace. Even if she isn't someone who wants to be in control, she can still enjoy the position if you take charge and move her around to suit you.

11. Edge of the Bed

This one is similar to the ankles up position in that it encourages deeper penetration. In the edge of the bed position, she lies on her back, and her hips are at the edge of the bed. You enter from under her legs. She can let them drop off the edge or rest them on your torso. Before you try this position, keep in mind the height of the bed and whether your groin will be in line with hers or not. You might need to bend or lower yourself a bit in order to penetrate her completely. The feel is sexy though because it suggests an urgency and impatience – as though you couldn't wait to get on to the bed properly. Not only that, she gets to view all the action, which, trust me, is hot!

12. Cowgirl with a Twist

Alright, so this is cowgirl but a bit more than just that. She assumes the cowgirl position, straddling you and facing your head. Then you raise your knees so as to support her bottom. She can, then, push off your chest and slide up and down against your thighs. Be warned, though – the lady controls when you climax so she can delay it if she wants. You want her to get there though so this shouldn't be a problem. To add spice, meet each of her thrusts by grabbing on to her thighs or hips.

13. The Bridge

So, this one starts out innocently enough with the missionary position. Then you need to sit up and ensure that your weight is supported on your ankles. Your knees need to be spread wide for balance. She should lie on her back with her feet flat on the bed. Then, she should arch her hips up so that she's in a low bridge position. This way you get the perfect angle for penetration and the maximum amount of penetration. If she finds the position uncomfortable, you can put some pillows under her back to prop it up.

14. Belly Down

Alright, this is a slightly new one compared to what we've discussed before and the sensations generated are new too. She goes on the bottom, face-down. You are on top either lying on top of her or utilizing a sort of a semi-push up position. Then you enter her. She needs to keep her legs straight and her hips slightly raised to facilitate the penetration. This works out great for both of you. Your penis is straight in line with her G-spot so you hit it on every thrust. She is super snug, so you get a great tight fit. Use a water based lube to ensure that everything glides into position as smoothly as possible. You can raise her hips by propping pillows under her pelvic region or vagina, especially if you're having a problem with alignment due to different heights.

15. Standing Against a Wall

This one is a classic quickie position. It is also one of oldest positions for a quickie. For it to work best, she needs to be the one against the wall. She needs to lean her pelvis forward, and her shoulders and back should be braced against the wall for support. Then she should wrap her leg around your waist. This controls your penetration and speed. The two requirements for this position to work out well are: the two partners should be of similar height, and she should have strong leg muscles. If there is a significant height difference, you may find it challenging to penetrate her.

16. Bent at the Waist

This one involves you standing behind her, while bends at the waist, as the name suggests and you enter her from behind. This position makes her vaginal walls tighter and therefore increases the friction. It doesn't hurt that this is an easy angle for penetration. Don't just expect her to bend without support, though – that could quickly become uncomfortable for her. Instead, ensure that there is something in front for her to hold on to such as a table, the back of a chair or a couch or even a sink. If she has that support, it leaves your hands free – you can use one hand to hold on to her and the other to reach around and rub her clitoris.

17. Missionary with a Twist

This one involves you getting into the missionary position and then, as the name says, turning onto your side – both of you. You need to use your arms to support each other and intertwine your legs so that you get a better fit and more leverage. You stay connected to each other the entire time. You move very slowly and roll to the side while still having intercourse. Of course, the clitoral stimulation doesn't let up which obviously is very important for her to reach the big O.

18. Cross-Legged

A common misconception about this position is that you need to be very flexible to be able to pull it off. While sitting in a cross-legged like a pretzel position is great, it's not necessary. All you really need is to sit cross legged so that your erection points upwards. She will sit facing you in your lap and wrap her legs around your waist or your hips. This works for both of you because you get maximum penetration while she controls the thrusts by riding or rocking. She can hold on to your shoulders for support.

19. The Spider

In this position, both of you need to be sitting on the bed, facing each other. Lean back on your hands for support. Your legs should be pointed towards one another. She needs to walk her feet over your body and to the sides of your hips and place her feet flat on the bed. This position allows you to penetrate her perfectly. Don't thrust into her; rock back and forth. The best part is that you can look at each other and at the action going on and she gets to control the motion, speed and angle to get to her climax.

20. The Pretzel

Again you don't have to be a flexible practitioner of the most difficult yoga that you can find to do this. This one is actually a mix of Doggy Style and face to face. She needs to lie down on her left side. Then you straddle her left leg, and she wraps her right leg around your waist. Feel free to determine what works best for both of you in this one.

So, I've listed twenty positions that guarantee pleasure not just for you but for her every time. Once you are comfortable with these positions, go ahead and experiment to see what works out best for both of you. Talk to each other about what worked and what didn't. If you find a position particularly difficult, try practicing with each other while fully clothed. Spontaneity is all well and good, but sometimes practice is better – after all, it does make perfect.

Chapter 6: Additional Tips To Help Both Of You Out

We've discussed techniques, positions and procedures. We've tried to understand the history of the female orgasm, what influences it and how to achieve it. While techniques and positions are great, remember that a woman orgasms as much from her mind as she does from her body. To help her get there, you need to ensure that her brain enjoys the experience as much as her body does. Here are some additional tips to help you get brain and body in sync and take her to the ultimate explosion.

Stop Worrying About Time

Your worry is about how long you may last. For her, the worry is about whether she's taking too long. As I've mentioned earlier, women do take longer to achieve an orgasm than do men. Having said that, it is very possible that she feels self-conscious about how long she's taking to get there and therefore ends up faking an orgasm rather than making it to the finish line.

To help her out with this one, take the pressure off her and yourself. Tell her that she and you have the whole night to get where both of you need to go. She needs to relax to be able to have an orgasm at all. So, let her do that and focus on the journey. Show her that not only are you in it for the long haul and that you like (as in really like) her sexual responses. The better she feels about this, the more likely she is to achieve climax.

Use Your Talent

Whatever it may be, it'll turn her on. Croon 'Careless Whisper' or show her your etchings (before you show her your 'etchings'). Studies at the Kinsey Institute show that talent is actually a greater turn on for women than chiseled abs or film-star good looks. If humor is your forte, use it. Connect with her on this level and she'll feel more comfortable with you and more attracted to you.

Tell Her What You Like About Her Body

Again, as I've mentioned earlier, body issues can become a great big roadblock on the way to orgasmic bliss for her. To reassure her and remove this roadblock, tell her what you like about her body. You don't have to make stuff up – after all, you do like her naked, right? Just tell her.

Be Gentle Up Top

More than the areola and the nipples, the top, bottom and sides of her breasts are sensitive. Gently brush your fingers, hands and lips on these areas. Pay close attention to her responses. Slowly build up to the nipples. Once the arousal builds, her nipples are ready for your attention and so is she.

Learn What Strokes Play Her Just Right

Remember, we women like a slow buildup. Hard and fast doesn't always work out so well for us. Here's a way you can build up the stimulation. Lying next to her, place the heel of one hand just above her clitoris. Next, you need to run your middle finger and your ring finger along her outer lips. Start with a feather touch and then build the pressure up. Use your palm to cup the area around her clitoris so that the sensation builds up. Don't try to touch the clitoris directly in the beginning. It's a sensitive bundle, and most women won't be ready for the sensation of direct stimulation. As her arousal builds up, you can brace your hand on her pubic mound or her mons and use the tips of your fingers to tease her clitoris while moving your hand.

Try a Different Angle

Tried and tested is fine for a while but make sure that you keep things fresh and interesting. Try different positions and different angles of penetration to see what works for her and you. Remember to use positions and angles that hit her G-spot every time. You can even use your fingers to massage the area. If a particular position or angle doesn't work for her, don't sweat it; just move on.

Multitasking is Hot

To ensure maximum pleasure for her, try out moves that bring you in contact with several of her sensitive zones at the same time. For example, you can have her lie on her back. She should stretch out her legs. Get on top and curl your arms around her shoulders. Use your elbows to support yourself and bring your chest level with her chin. This is another way you can achieve the oft-mentioned and very successful coital alignment technique.

Watch Out for Signs of Her Orgasm

When you start oral sex, don't go hell for leather right from the outset. Remember, gentle and slow build up is the key here. Don't even start with her vagina. Try her hips and then move to her thighs and then her inner thighs. Different women are sensitive in different parts so figure that out. Then move to her outer and inner lips and kiss them. Finally, move inside using broad and firm strokes of your tongue.

Throughout all of this, watch and listen to determine what she likes and what she loves. Listen to her moans and cries. See how her hips move. You can tell when she's close to orgasm by the changing color of her labia, which happens because of increased blood flow. You can also put your hand on her stomach to check for the contractions that happen immediately before her orgasm.

Follow Her Lead

This is where things are different for men and women. When you start on the road to your climax, nothing and I mean nothing will derail you (short of the possibility of Lorena Bobbitt appearing in your bedroom). Unfortunately, the same is not true for your lady. While changing positions midway to the big O might not affect your arousal, it could ring the death knell for hers. Try new things; just not when she's about to explode. The whole thing will end up a complete anti-climax for her (pun definitely intended).

Let the Lady Go First

Be a gentleman here and let her hit her orgasm first. While it's great that you want both of you to come together, let's face it, that doesn't always work out. Chances are you'll hit the goal first, and she'll be left far behind in your wake. Too much rubbing of the clitoris can even desensitize it, killing any chance of her achieving an orgasm. So, ensure she has come at least once before intercourse.

An added bonus here is that once she's come for the first time, her orgasm threshold will drop. This means that it's easier for you to bring her to climax a second or a third time.

Chapter 7: Myths About Female Orgasms

Unfortunately, despite a much more open attitude towards female sexuality and orgasms than society has had in the past, there are plenty of myths still doing the rounds. A lot of information out there is bad or compared to male orgasms which actually happen very differently. In this chapter, I'll undertake the busting of some of these myths and hope that you, my gentlemen readers, are not led astray by them.

1.   Orgasm is the End Goal of Sex

No, no and a thousand times no. My vehemence about this point is because it puts too much pressure on both the partners to achieve and help each other achieve orgasm. An activity that is really about pleasure and intimacy becomes a race to the finish. Instead, take time out to explore each other (ladies, I'm looking at you too) and learn what works for both of you. Try out something new or just a variation of something tried and tested. Take pleasure in being with each other, even if this is something you've done a gazillion times before.

2.   Multiple Orgasms Are Easy for All Women

Nope, not true. Yes, we do have the capacity for multiple orgasms (lucky us). But most women actually don't have them, regardless of what the movies say. Even the women who do have them don't achieve them easily and don't have them every time. Typically, women who have multiple orgasms have trained themselves, or their partners, to hit their pleasure spots just right every time. This is not something that will just happen, so give her and yourself some time to learn what works for both of you.

### 3.	All Women like Romantic Movie Sex

Umm, not always. While gentle and tender is nice, we like getting it hard and rough too (find out before you try it though). Sometimes, the mood is just not right for romance, but it is right for hard, pure sex. We do enjoy that just as much as men do, you know.

### 4.	Safer Sex Isn't Sexier Sex

Ok, this one is just plain crazy. We think ourselves into orgasms, remember? Do you really think a woman will be able to come if she's worrying about a potential baby or a sexually transmitted infection or disease? Besides, you using protection shows us you care about our safety and well-being, and that is sexy.

### 5.	Skilled Partner Means No Sex Toys

Actually, a partner is skilled if he knows how to bring a woman to a climax. As such, using sex toys to maximize her pleasure actually shows off his skill. His mad skills and toys both? Ooh la la!

6.   All Women Can Orgasm Easily

All I'm going to say about this one is that if this statement were true, this e-book wouldn't be necessary.

7.   Penetration is Needed For a Woman to Orgasm

As the techniques discussed in this book shows, this one is simply not true. Clitoral stimulation is what leads to female orgasm most of the time, and penetration is not needed to stimulate a woman's clitoris. Since there are different types other than a penetration orgasm, we'll just leave it at that.

8.   You will go blind or hair will grow on your palms

This was created in order to shame people so that they would not please themselves because it made them think that they were going to end up with a physical deformity. However, as we can tell from thousands of years of people pleasing themselves, this is a complete lie!

9.   If you orgasm while masturbating, you cannot orgasm while having actual sex.

As long as you do not allow for your masturbation schedule to get in the way of having orgasms with your partner, then you have nothing to worry about! In fact, when you are having sex with your partner and trying to reach that glorious end, you can use toys or masturbation during sex in order to climax if you are having trouble.

10. **You are in a relationship, you do not need to be masturbating.**

Well, masturbating is actually been found to help women show their partner's what it is that they like for when their partners go to touch them. And as we just mentioned, touching yourself during sex can actually assist in bringing on your orgasm. And last but not least, do people think that you are going to just sit around and wait for sex if your partner is out of town? I wouldn't! Why not spice things up and touch yourself while you are on the phone with your partner? It will definitely help with the orgasm when your partner does return because they know exactly what they have been missing!

Chapter 8: Solo Play

Sometimes when push comes to shove you have to take things into your own hands. Solo paly is going to be the best way for you to be able to tell your partner how you like it and how to reach your orgasm!

When you are playing alone, you can use your hands or toys whichever way you find that you are going to be able to find that you are reaching your final destination. Sometimes, it also helps to make up fantasies when you are doing solo play because it is going to give you something to focus on, such as that hot actor's hands all over your body in ways that no one else has ever touched you before!

Masturbation tips

1. Get into the mood! Nothing is worse than when you are trying to get off and you find that you are not in the mood. So, making sure that you are in the proper mood is going to be the number one thing. However, only you are going to know if you are in the mood for your play time or not.

    Some people do not take much to get into the mood, all they need to do is pull out the toys or lay in bed. Other people have to drag it out and make it elaborate so that they feel special before they are able to start.

2. Privacy. Nothing is more embarrassing than someone walking in on what you are doing! It is the fastest way

for a mood to be killed. So, no matter where you are, make sure that you can lock the door so that no one is coming in on you. If you do not feel comfortable masturbating when there are other people in the house, then you should wait till there is no one there and you are going to have a little bit of time to yourself in order to allow yourself time to be vocal.

It is also a good idea to keep your phone off, on silent, or even in the other room so that it is not breaking your concentration.

3. Focus on your clitoris. As you are working on your solo play, you are going to come to realize that having a clitoral orgasm is going to be a lot easier to achieve than a vaginal orgasm. This is especially going to help when you are first learning how to masturbate.

The first thing that you need to know is that your clitoris is the small bundle of nerves that gets bigger the more aroused that you are. It can be located above your vagina and under a small fold of skin that will be extremely sensitive after you have found your climax.

When you are wanting to stimulate your clit, you are going to rub it with your fingers. For some women, this is the best way to get your orgasm. But, others find that it is going to give them more stimulation by using indirect stimulation so they do not touch it directly, they rub around it to make it more sensitive. You may want to massage it slowly before you begin to get rough with it so that you are able to build your climax up and so that you are getting your body use to a new source of stimulation.

4. Gspots are another great way to have an orgasm. Sadly, many people do not know where their gspot is because it is only going to be found when it is engorged which is going to happen when you are aroused.

    The gspot is going to be located inside of your vagina on the front wall. It is going to be slightly rough to the touch but it is going to be similar to running your tongue across the top of your mouth.

    Gspot stimulation comes in many different forms such as inserting your fingers into your vagina and curling them into a come-hither motion thus allowing your fingers to press against it. From there, you are going to be able to masturbate how you find comfortable. Other ways are to use toys but the toys are going to be your own decision because what works for you may not work for your best friend.

5. Lube. It may seem a little out there to use lube when you are masturbating but lube is not just to use with another person. there are different types of lubes that are going to amp up that pleasurable feeling. You are going to have to experiment to find out which lube is right for you.

6. Toys toys everywhere! If all else fails, one of the best ways to make your orgasm more intense is to use toys.

There are many different toys that are on the market and the one that works best for you is the one that you are going to find that you cannot live without.

For many, a vibrator is all that they need because they are able to adjust the speed and place the pulsing toy next to their clit or in their vagina and find that perfect spot that sends them towards a screaming oh. However, you have to be careful with some vibrators because they tend to get stuck at a high speed and then become too strong.

Dildos are another option and are great for whenever your partner is not there. Some dildos even going to double as a vibrator and can reach places that fingers never will be able to.

Last but not least, you can use a butt plug. There are some women in the world that have said having something in their behind make their orgasm more intense. This is not going to be true for every woman, but it is going to be true for some.

7. Porn is not just for guys. For some porn gives the proper images and noises that make it to where you are able to find your orgasm. Sometimes you do not have to watch it, just the noises help. But, there are all variations of porn out there and you have to find what works best for you.

8. Erotic stories are going to allow you to create your own images. But they are not going to be for

everyone. If you do not find anything else that works, this is one thing to try.

9. Keep learning!! There is always more that you can learn about your body and masturbation. Pick up a book, search online and you will find what you are looking for that works for you.

Techniques to use when you are masturbating

1. Up and down: this one is pretty easy and it is going to focus mainly on your clit. Take however many fingers you want to use and rub up and down beside your clit. If you are wanting more simulation, you can rub your clit directly.

2. Long slow stroke: still using your fingers, you are going to go from the middle of your clit to the bottom of your vagina. You are going to find which areas of your vagina make you jerk and which ones your body does not like. do not ignore your body and do things that your body does not like or you are not going to reach your orgasm.

3. Side to side: just like when you were going up and down, on your clit. But this time you are going to go side to side. When you are using this technique you can also include

    a. Switching directions

    b. Using indirect contact

c. Different speeds

d. The number of fingers that you use

e. The pressure you are using

f. Lube

4. Fun with four fingers: you are going to use four fingers to go over your clit in order to stimulate your climax. You are going to hold your four fingers togheer and rub them around your clit and vagina. You can do circles or you can go side to side depending on what you prefer. This is also going to stimulate your uspot.

5. Uspot: your uspot is going to be slightly lower than your clit and is above the urethral opening. When you are wanting to stimulate it, you will stroke it with just the tip of your finger. The softer that you rub it along with rubbing your clit, the more stimulation you are going to experience.

6. Shower head love: do not be afraid to admit it, using the shower head or the faucet is a great way to get off. If you have yet to do it, then you are going to want to get to it because it is one of the best methods to use for masturbation!

    You are not going to have to use your fingers if you do not want to and you are going to be able to get the entirety of your vagina so that you can find the perfect spot. With the shower head, you can change the pressure of the water, how far away it is from your vagina, or the temperature of the water to find your orgasm.

7. Under the hood: you may or may not have noticed that you have a clitoris that is super sensitive. Not all women have this, but when it is sensitive, it can sometimes be pleasurable to touch so you have to find other ways to masturbate.

    One of the methods that you can use is to use the hood of your clitoris as a butter so that you are not touching your clitoris directly.

8. Hood life: there are other women whose clit is not sensitive at all and they have to move the hood of their clitoris. Women like this usually have to rub and grind in order to get their clitoris stimulated. Instead, you can always move the hood and get straight to your clitoris without any harm.

9. Orgasmic mediation: for this technique, you are going to lay on your back and spready our legs so that they are not harming you, but you can easily get to your vagina. You are then going to stroke your clitoris and various other parts of your vagina.

    You can also do this with a partner and have your partner sit to your right with his left leg over your stomach holding you down slightly with his other leg under your right leg.

10. The squeeze: when using the squeeze, you are going to be focusing on your clitoris. The first thing that you are going to do is place your thumb and index finger on either side of your clit. From there you are going to squeeze starting with a gentle pressure and upping the pressure until you are able to stimulate your clit into an orgasm.

11. Lovely Labia: as you rub on your labia it is a good source of foreplay and if done right, you will achieve an orgasm. Some ways you can add to rubbing your labia are:

    a. Running different materials over it

    b. Run your fingers up and down it

    c. Use lube for a silky feeling.

    d. Squeeze your fingers together.

12. Use a pillow: some women like to hump or grind in order to get their orgasm. Things like toys, blankets, and pillows are good for this technique so you can stimulate your clitoris and labia at the same time.

    a. Use your partner's thigh

b. Lie on your side with a pillow between your legs. Squeezing your legs together, and pull the pillow between your legs so it is pressing against all your gooey parts before beginning to grind

c. Put a towel over your pillow and grind on that so that you get a different feeling. Not only are you keeping your pillow dry, but you can try other things like toys or electric toothbrushes.

d. A small pillow can be folded in half to achieve the same effect if you do not have a long pillow.

13. Pearl necklace: when doing pearl necklace, you will take beads of some sort between your legs. You will lay on your back and place the beads so that they are across your entire vagina. You will pull the beads up and down slowly to stimulate yourself. Some lube on the beads makes it to where you are not having such a rough surface.

You can also use a towel or silk scarf for this method. However, do not use anything too expensive just in the event it breaks.

14. Vibrators are great if you cannot get any of these methods to work. There are so many kinds of vibrators out there that you are going to have to experiment and find the one that works best for you. There are vibrators that are no bigger than the tip of your finger and then there are ones that you have to

plug into the wall. But in the end, they are all going to give you the explosion that you want.

If you are too scared to go to a sex toy store that is in your area, you are able to order them offline. However, when you order offline you are not going to be able to tell if that is the proper one for you. Getting a feel for the vibrator is part of what tells you if it is the one for you or not.

Ultimately, there are several different ways that you are going to be able to get off when you are masturbating, it is up to you to find the way that works best. If you want to masturbate while your partner watches, then that is completely your choice because this is about you! Go on and get your orgasm because you deserve it!

Chapter 9: Getting the Best Orgasm of Your Life

- Getting off can sometimes be hard because of things that get in the way such as muscle cramps! However, if you are wanting to experience that mystical gem that is known as the multiple orgasms, or even just get your first orgasm, there are a few things that you are going to want to know so that you can get the best orgasm of your life.

- Coregasms: there is always more than one way to get to your orgasm and the path that you choose is going to be the one that is best for you. However, one thing that most people do not understand is that you can reach your orgasm by exercising! Research has proven that some women have an orgasm by having pelvic muscle contractions and tightening up their legs and abdominal muscles as they are working out. Having an orgasm and losing weight? Sign me up!

- Birthgasms: it does not happen to many, but there have been some women that find an orgasm when they are in the middle of labor. Like we just mentioned, it is the tightening of those abdominal muscles and the pelvic contractions that lead you to it. But, think about who you have in the birthing room just in case this happens to you. There is nothing more embarrassing than getting off in front of your mother in law.

- Thoughts: it has been found that the correct amount of visualization, giving yourself permission, and counting will allow you to have an orgasm in their own head. It is a great way to practice your orgasms so that you can achieve them when you are in bed.

- Volume: adding in things like high pitched noises or low pitch can also affect your orgasm. The high-pitched noises are going to increase the sexual energy that is coursing through your head, chest, and throat. Obviously, the pitches are going to impact your lower half and bring you to that magical moment.

- Pillow talk: meeting your end releases oxytocin in your brain which makes your emotions heightened. Depending on whole you just got done doing the nasty with depends on if you want to have pillow talk. If it is just a random hook up, stick to the spooning so you are not saying something you regret later on.

Every woman is not the same! So, what works for one will not work for another all the time. Not to mention your nationality is going to play a part in how many times you do the nasty.

Conclusion

So here we are at the end of the journey. I hope that you gentlemen have learned more about women and their orgasms and feel more confident about being able to please your partners. You should now be aware of how the female orgasm has been perceived throughout history. You also know the factors that affect the ability of a woman to achieve an orgasm during sexual intercourse.

I hope you now understand the different types of orgasms women can have and how you can ensure that they receive them. If you go through the fifteen-minute quickie guide, it can actually act as a blueprint for pretty much all of your sexual encounters, no matter how much time you intend to take over them. All that varies is how much time you would spend on each of the steps I've outlined. Remember to switch things up, because variety is the spice of life! It'll keep your sex life happy and interesting long after your first encounter with your partner. The different positions I've outlined in Chapter 5 should help both of you enjoy a great time in bed and out of it. Just keep in mind that it is all about the journey and not the destination. Take pleasure in each other and in giving each other pleasure and the orgasms will take care of themselves.

I've also added a few tips that I think you will find useful, not only in terms of physical stimulation but also in terms of mental reassurance and comfort. Women's orgasms are as much a product of their minds as of their bodies. Remember to keep the mind as relaxed as possible so that the body can enjoy the sexual act. Listen to the cues your partner gives you, both verbal and physical and use those to determine what works for her and what doesn't.

I hope that you enjoyed this book and took away something useful from it. If you would be willing to leave a review about this book, I would be very grateful. Thank you very much for purchasing and reading my book. I wish you many healthy, safe and happy sexual encounters.

Introduction Book 2

The following chapters will discuss how to make your sex life with your man the best it could possibly be. While sex is definitely a game that is played between the sheets (or against the wall or over the table or in a dungeon or wherever you'd legally like), much of what goes on between those sheets also goes on between your ears and between your emotions. This ebook will cover several different subjects to ensure that not only are you the best he's ever had but he keeps on coming back for more again and again!

We'll work on the emotional component of sex and how to connect with your man on a deeper level. We'll also discuss some differences between men and women in this arena. We'll move on to talk about the mentality of sex and how to get your minds into the act as much as your bodies. Finally, we will, of course, talk about the physicality of sex and ensure that you're the best he'll never forget. This book also addresses your pleasure, as well! Sex should be fun for both (or all) parties involved in it and we're here to give you the tools necessary to make that happen.

There are plenty of books on this subject on the market, thanks again for choosing this one! Every effort was made to ensure it is full of as much useful information as possible, please enjoy!

Part 1: A Mental Introduction to Your Man

One of the most overlooked components of sex is the mind, unfortunately. Of course, when you think "sex organs" you probably don't think "brain" right away, but you definitely should! What your man thinks about sex will translate to the reality of sex, and understanding how his mind works will give you a big boost when it comes to the horizontal tango.

Chapter 1: What do Men Really Think About Sex?

If you think *men and sex* you likely believe that your man wants sex all day, every day, and all the time. In reality, this is not true. Men can be *in the mood* or *out of the mood* just as much as you can, and for just as many reasons. We've surveyed several men anonymously when it comes to their opinions on sex and they've given us the following:

The players don't mind getting played. Most men are *actually very happy* to get played by women. That's right. The bad boys like bad girls themselves. *This* is why so many women end up wondering why good guys end up with girls that treat them badly. It's *entirely possible* to have a man that is so wrapped around your finger that they'll turn their head away from your every flaw. Most men we surveyed weren't exactly proud to admit this, but most have had an experience with a woman like this at least once in their lives. One man described it as "being under a magic spell." So you've got a lot of power in your sexuality, ladies!

It's not just about how hot you are. While no man we surveyed would turn down a 10/10 if she approached him at a bar, all of the men said that good looks and tight bodies are not nearly enough for a satisfying sex life. In fact, a good portion of the men we sampled said that they would actually prefer less pure physical attraction for more mental and emotional connection. Sex is also about the environment. This doesn't necessarily mean you need to light your house up like a candle factory every time you want to get down; however, the ambiance can affect a man's libido.

Objectification is going to be the name of the game. Many of the more egalitarian men we surveyed reported feeling guilty about having a desire to objectify women, but the sheer beauty of the feminine made it difficult for some to believe that women existed on the same planet as them. While men may read feminist literature and truly believe in the equality of the sexes on a daily basis, the sheer raw power of female sexuality makes many men elevate females to the level of goddesses.

If you want to have sex with them, they likely will have sex with you. Of course, there are mitigating factors, here - many men report married women being a no-go (for likely obvious reasons) and most men say that they would remain loyal if married themselves. *However*, if you are at a bar and

you want to have sex with the man that you're talking to…
your chances are extremely good. Most men are extremely
flattered when a woman wants to have sex with them, so
even if they aren't particularly attracted to you, most will be
down to clown regardless. Even in the event that a man is
resistant for a period of time… if you're persistent enough
your chances are pretty good. This is *not* an excuse to harass
men; it's just another example of how very powerful your
feminine charms are.

Get into penis worship. Men love it when a woman is
thrilled to interact with their penis. Even though many men
don't like to admit it, *most* are very attached to their dicks.
(Even beyond the fact that the dick is a part of his body.)
They don't just want a woman to have sex with… they want
a woman's eyes to alight with pleasure before going down
for a blowjob. If you want to blow a man out of the water,
do it by being excited about his Johnson.

Men do care if you orgasm. It's a popular trope that men
just like to jackhammer away, but this is absolutely not
true… but perhaps not for the nicest reasons in the world.
Men care about making women orgasm because it makes
them feel good. Giving somebody else pleasure is a power
trip, and men love that almost as much as they love
orgasming themselves.

Keep in mind that these thoughts are *solely* about sex and
not about love. But this information should be pretty
powerful for you and may give you a deeper insight into
how the male mind perceives sex. If nothing else, be aware
of how much power you have over the men, ladies!

Chapter 2: How To Think Like a Man

Now that you've gotten a glimpse into the mind of your average man when it comes to sex, it's also important to understand how men work in general. While men and women are actually both from Earth and not from Mars and Venus, there are some serious differences between the sexes that you need to be aware of. The more that you know about your man, the better your chances are of getting what you want out of him.

Men don't over think it. Women are constantly searching for the connections between everything and trying to figure out the *why*, particularly when it comes to interpersonal interaction. *Why didn't he text me back right away? Why did he text a smiley emoji with his 'hi'? Why hasn't he introduced me to his mother yet?*

Women are programmed to figure out the *why* and with men, the why is often as simple as the word *because*. Why didn't he text you back right away? Likely because he simply didn't think of it. Why did he use the smiley emoji? Because it was the first one that popped up when he accidentally hit the emoji button. Why hasn't he introduced you to his mother? It hasn't come up.

Men are a lot simpler than many women make them out to be. It's *women* who tend to overcomplicate the dance between the sexes, not men.

Men have a language, and that language is *obvious*. Many women waste a lot of time at the bars trying to drop *hints* to a man that she wants him to go over and talk to her. The trouble with this is that men *suck* at picking up hints. Men speak the language of *obvious*.

It really is a shame that the gender roles in our culture have reduced us to sending smoke signals that the other sex has no idea how to interpret or pick up on. If you want a man to talk to you at the bar, *go talk to the man*. As we've already discussed, the simple fact that a woman wants to have sex with a man will often be enough to make the man have sex with her on its own.

A woman at a bar who makes the first move on a man is very likely to get the man's attention very quickly. Because you're speaking his language.

Men *like* it when women are obvious. Men adore it when they can actually tell what your intentions are. Most of the time, they are not sitting around and thinking about how easy you must be if you're batting your eyelashes at them too often or whatever you're worried about.

Men love it when the tables are turned and women approach them. In fact, many men we talked to said that the fantasy of an aggressive woman was extremely hot. Even those who prefer their women more mild-mannered said that they would definitely enjoy being bought a drink at the bar. Basically, ladies, if you want to communicate effectively with your man, you need to communicate *obviously* with them.

Men are very literal creatures overall and will react *well* to you being open with your desire for them.

This also translates directly to the bedroom! If you want to have sex, make it be known! This will put him on the moon, that you're being the proactive one in the relationship. Men love this and absolutely crave it.

Chapter 3: How to Communicate With Your Man

Let's talk a little bit more about how best to communicate with your man. We've discussed that being *obvious* is very important to men, but more advisable to never hurt when attempting to win the battle of the sexes!

Make no assumptions whatsoever. So let's assume that you take the advice from the previous chapter and decide to go with *obvious*. The trouble is that what is *obvious* to you may not be *obvious* to him. (The course of true love never did run smooth.)

For example, let's say that you want your man to be more affectionate toward you. So you say, "Honey, I need you to be more affectionate." This is definitely obvious, but the only thing that's obvious is that you *need something*.

So don't just tell your man that you want something out of him. Tell him *specifically* what you want. If *affection* to you means more hugs or more texts or more gifts or a different kind of sex or *whatever* you need, tell him that specifically. Don't make vague demands. You will get a muddled response at best and your man will be frustrated if he can't make you happy.

Be positive. Particularly if you are talking about something you are unhappy about, you'll get much farther with men if you couch it in positive language. For example, "I really have fun with you when we go out on the town - can we go out this Friday?" will likely get a much better response than, "Why don't you take me out anymore?"

The first one is a fun and playful request that will likely get an eager response - your man probably likes to go out and have fun with you as well. The *second* one just sounds like whining. Plus, in the first response, you are being obvious and proactive. You're saying that you want something (you want to go out with him and have fun), and then you're saying exactly what you want to do (go out this Friday). The second statement sounds like you're handing him a problem that is *his fault* and he has to fix it.

Both sentences mean the same thing. One will get a better response than the other.

Be truthful. One of the things that drive men crazy about women is that many women seem to expect men to be mind readers. One of the worst phrases a man can hear is, "Don't worry, it's nothing," when he is perfectly aware that *something* is afoot.

What makes this even worse is that in the event that the man takes the woman at her *word* that there is no problem… most of the time the woman will get angry at the man for not divining the fact that there actually *is* a problem. This is a negative loop that will definitely hurt your relationship. If there is a problem, tell your man that there is a problem.

Keep positive and constructive and it is likely you will find a solution.

Actively listen. Men talk too. Men articulate their feelings and desires, and you need to listen to those as much as he needs to listen to you. Particularly if you are having an argument, it is important to stay present in the moment and ensure that you are actively listening to what your partner has to say. Many times in an argument people will start constructing what they want to say in response before their partner stops speaking.

This is bad because then nobody feels heard. Make sure to actively listen to your man, even when you don't agree with him. This will help ensure that he feels heard and ensure that the argument can be solved and doesn't snowball into something bigger.

Let him talk for himself and say it his way. Many women have a tendency to interrupt their mates in an attempt to better *interpret* what they're saying and restate it. This can be dangerous, particularly if you are misunderstanding what your partner is saying.

Actively listen, and let your man speak for himself. This will not only help him feel heard but also respected and not like you're trying to put words in his mouth. Plus, if you're not letting him speak for yourself, you could end up projecting your frustrations onto him and this will end up hurting your relationship and your sex life.

Chapter 4: Why to Fuck His Mind Before You Fuck his Body

Much of this section of the book didn't even talk about sex that much, but the reality is that the brain is probably the biggest sex organ of all if taken in the long run.

Of course, if you're just having a one-night stand, focusing *too* much on communication issues may actually hurt you more than help you. But if you're looking to build a sexual relationship with your man that will stand the test of time and absolutely blow him out of the water, it's important to fuck his mind before you fuck his body.

Having sex with your mind makes the entire experience of sex that much more intimate. Sex, when taken at its most basic level, is simply biology. We are biologically wired to mate, and the majority of humanity is biologically wired to mate with the opposite sex.

However, *good* sex is much more than this. It's not simply just the ability to stick a penis in a vagina and have done with it. *Truly* good sex comes from a meeting of the minds.

So, here's a question - *do* you want to meet your guy's mind and does he want to meet yours, or are you simply on the physical level? There's nothing wrong with a quick fuck, but if you want to really make sex mean something and deliver mind-blowing pleasure for both parties, you also have to want to intellectually fuck the other person.

What's your relationship like with your man? Do you enjoy talking to each other about non-sex related subjects? Do you find his mind as sexy as you find his body?

You need to be able to respect each other's opinions in order to work. Many a relationship has been wrecked by completely different spiritual or political beliefs. It's important to understand your overall views on life before investing too much time into any relationship.

You will also want to talk about your sexual desires. Is either one of you kinky or do you both prefer the mechanics of vanilla sex? If one of you is a kinkster and the other is completely vanilla, that will cause issues in the long term as well.

Again, you want to be able to understand and respect your partner's mind. Once you have this mental connection, the sex is sure to be out-of-this-world.

Part 2: Connect With Your Man's Emotions

Not to get too mushy on you, but sex isn't just about mind and body - it's about emotions, too. And while you may be hung up on the traditional image of the emotionless masculine male, nothing could be more false. Men have emotions to0… just as many as you do. You may express them differently and you might feel them slightly differently, but they certainly exist.

If you want to fuck his brains out, you're going to need to understand him on an emotional level.

Chapter 5: Male Emotions vs. Female Emotions

The traditional wisdom says that women are naturally programmed to be more emotional than men. However, science suggests that this is likely not the case, because men and women do seem to process emotional stimuli differently.

A study was conducted where roughly 4,000 men and women were exposed to images that contained varying kinds of emotional content. For example, some of the photos were happy images (like a child playing with a puppy), some of them were negative images (like people crying at a funeral) and others were emotionally neutral (like a picture of a building in a city).

After being exposed to the images, researchers asked the participants about the content of the images.

Women were more likely to rate pictures as emotional overall and were more likely to react to negative imagery than men were. However, both men and women reacted in the same way to the neutral images.

Participants also engaged in a memory test, asking if they were able to recall the images or not. Women were able to recall significantly more images than the men were, particularly in the case of the positive images.

MRI data suggested that women experienced greater stimuli in the brain as compared to men. Certain areas of the brain were stimulated in women who looked at the images that were not stimulated in the brains of men.

Outside of this study, other studies have suggested that women display a more visual reaction to negative stimuli than men do.

So, in this case, the literal brain activity of men and women are different. Women tend to react more strongly to emotional images and also have a greater recollection of emotional experiences than men do. In essence, women tend to experience stronger impact from emotions than men do.

Researchers are still unsure if this is more the result of *nurture or nature,* however, there are many societal expectations on men not to show emotion nor react to it as much as women do. For instance, it is much more socially acceptable for women to cry in public as compared to men.

So this doesn't mean that your man doesn't have emotions. *He does.* You just need to understand how he may express them differently than you do. His physical and mental reaction to emotions will not be the same as yours, but he still *has them.*

If you want to make sex an incredible and meaningful experience, you need to unlock the power of his emotions.

Chapter 6: How to Make a Man Feel Safe

In order for men to share their emotions with you, you are going to need to make him feel safe enough to do so. Men are taught to hide their emotions from nearly everybody, including their friends. Men do not talk about their emotional lives with their friends as much as women do, in 99% of cases. So if you want to break this barrier, you're going to have to work for it.

Create the right environment for it. If you want a man to trust you with his emotions, you're going to need to create an environment where he feels safe to share them with you. This will have a lot to do with your reactions to him.

Men are going to be more willing to open up to you if they believe that they won't be judged or criticized for it. You can hint that you're the woman that he can confide in by showing your appreciation for the things he does and not criticizing him. Of course, this doesn't mean that you should act as though he does no wrong (he definitely does, from time to time), but try and focus on the positives, as suggested earlier in the book.

For example, if he suggests a restaurant that turns out to be a total bomb, don't complain incessantly about how bad the experience was. He will feel responsible for it because *he* was the one that suggested the restaurant. Instead, try focusing on how nice it was that he wanted to go out with you and how much you appreciated his effort. This will show that even when he does things that don't result in a perfect ending, you'll still appreciate his thoughtfulness and who he is.

If your man believes that he does things correctly with you and is doing a good job in moving your relationship along, he will open up to you more and be more comfortable with you. Men are very sensitive to criticism, *especially* criticism from women.

Be open yourself. Again, women are traditionally expected to be the emotional ones in a relationship. If you come off like an ice queen to your man, he is likely not going to open himself up much in turn.

This doesn't mean that you have to cry all over him (and you probably shouldn't on the first date), but there are certain things it's okay to be open about. Are you nervous about the first date? Tell him! He'll like having the opportunity to try and reassure you. It will also make him feel a bit less pressured overall on the emotional front.

If you are open with him, it is more likely that he will be open with you. You may be surprised at how quickly your man will open up to you if you simply tell him the truth about your own emotions. There are *many* men out there who feel emotionally isolated.

Don't feel the need to control the entire relationship. Many women have a tendency to daydream about their forever relationship, where they get married to the man they're with and have babies and the picket fence and all of that.

While it's completely okay to have marriage and children as a life goal, try to avoid putting the relationship on the fast track toward that. This will likely alarm your man and make it even more difficult for you to be intimate around each other. He'll be concerned about you overwhelming him.

Take your time! Be in the present! Enjoy all of the little magical moments that you have with your man whether you're at a terrible restaurant or going to see a show or just sitting at home and watching Netflix. Take your time, and you'll be amazed at what you can get out of your man and how comfortable he'll become around you. *This* is the foundation for the forever relationships (and for great sex)!

Chapter 7: How to Create Emotional Intimacy with Your Man

If you want to create emotional intimacy, you need to lay the groundwork and actually see how he is *responding* to it. If you've been reading this book, you've likely figured out that creating this environment fertile to emotional intimacy is a lot of work.

But how do you know if he's responding the way you want? It can be difficult.

When you voice your emotions to your partner, how does he react?
If you are upset or angry or happy or nervous, you should put these feelings to direct words. Again, expecting him to read your mind is a one-way ticket to disaster.

However, when you voice your feelings… how does he react? Does he react with positive affirmations, or at least acknowledgement? Or does he seem disinterested? In healthy emotional relationships, partners at least acknowledge each other's feelings, even if they don't agree with them. If your man seems distant or completely uninterested in what you're feeling, that's a danger sign.

On the flipside, if you want to create an environment of emotional intimacy, you need to acknowledge when your man speaks to you about his emotions. Many men love it when their female partners act as an emotional sounding board. It makes them feel loved and appreciated.

Communicate directly with him. Again. Do not hint. If you want to spend more time with your man, do not attempt to do this by making him *jealous* by flirting with other men at the bar. This sends mixed signals and will absolutely not get you the response that you want.

If you express yourself in a clear and positive manner, you will get the results you want. Likewise, don't take his truthfulness as a personal attack. If you ask him how that dress looks on you and he doesn't like the dress… don't fly off the handle at him about it. You asked, and he responded. It doesn't mean he thinks you are unattractive. He simply didn't like the dress.

If you can engage in clear and constructive conversation and criticism of each other, it will actually deepen your intimacy because both of you know that your opinions are safe with each other.

Accept him and do not try to change him. Women are notorious for trying to mold their men into perfect relationship-material, and *this does not work.* The only person that you can change is yourself. Of course, there are some examples to this. If your man is a smoker and he decides that he wishes to quit, you can absolutely emotionally support him through being weaned off nicotine.

However, in this example, you are *helping* your man change in a way that he has decided on his own to do. If he doesn't want to quit smoking, demanding that he stop because *you* want him to is ineffective. Either accept that your man smokes cigarettes, or consider it a deal breaker and move on.

This also goes with emotions. If you tell your man that you really, really like him and he changes the subject or looks uncomfortable or otherwise does not respond with the same amount of affection that you do… do not try to get him to "love you more." This has to happen at its own pace. If it isn't happening, it isn't.

Likewise, if you want to create that awesome environment of intimacy, you definitely need to reciprocate his own displays of affection! If he tells you he loves you or adores you or wants you, make sure to tell him back in kind if you feel the same way!

Be open about sex. Obviously, if you want to fuck his brains out you need to be open and engaged with sex. However, it's important to figure out how both you and he react to each other in this manner. Do you feel inhibited or shy when bringing something up to him that you desire sexually? Are you hoping that sex will actually translate into him spending more time with you or giving you the affection that you crave?

Sex should be about sex alone. It is not a weapon that should be used to hurt your man, and it's not an item that should be exchanged for other commodities like love. You also should feel free to talk to your partner about your sexual desires. Of course, different people have different sexual desires - some may feel that mild bondage is extremely kinky, while others already have a dungeon set up in their basement for play.

The idea is not that you and your man can't have limits on what you will or won't do during sex, but that you are okay with talking about sex and you don't feel as though you'll be judged for bringing up things that you desire. For instance, some people couldn't imagine a sex life without anal, while others find the entire concept disgusting. For a great sex life, you need to be compatible in this manner.

Chapter 8: You're Not All That Different

Much of this part has focused heavily on the emotional differences between men and women, but the reality is that you are not that different from your man at the end of the day. They way that you express your emotions may be different, but both of you are humans and are both parts of the human experience.

While women are the ones that are typically stereotyped as emotional and clingy after sex, for instance, science suggests that this is not the case.

For instance, men are just as prone to experience some post-sex sadness the way that women are, even in the event that the encounter had nothing bad about it.

The evidence suggests that higher levels of testosterone may account for post-sex blues because higher testosterone levels lead to more negative communication after sex. Higher levels of testosterone tend to be found in people who didn't orgasm after sex.

Women tend to orgasm less during sex than men do, which could explain why women are reported to feel this way more often after sex than men. If you want to ensure that you beat the post-sex blues, communicate with your man and ensure that you're orgasming!

But men feel this way, too. Men report it less often, but researchers surmise that this is largely an omission issue, meaning that many men may feel sad after sex, but don't admit it.

You are not that different.

Chapter 9: Blow His Mind Physically

Now that we've talked about the mind and the emotions, let's get down to the nitty-gritty of how to *actually physically* blow his mind and be the best lay that he's ever had. This may be the easiest part (and the most fun), particularly if you've got a mental and emotional connection going on.

Sex is about fun and abandon. Probably the number one tip that you can get about six is simply to enjoy yourself. If you're not enjoying the sex, your partner will be able to tell and it will boomerang back onto him. So get out there, get in the sack, and have a hell of a time!

Chapter 9: Give the Best Blowjob Ever

All right. Let's get down to brass tacks and start talking about the BJ.

First of all, while it's not 100% necessary to give blow jobs in order to have great sex, the *vast vast majority of men* desire blowjobs. If you refuse to give your man a blowjob, there's a high likelihood that you won't be his girl for very long.

However, there are several tips for the squeamish. If you are concerned about unpleasant odors or tastes, suggest taking a shower before sex. He will very likely not say no and will certainly not say no to you soaping up his genitals. Then you can be assured he's as clean as can be.

Plus, don't feel as though you have to *swallow*, (and if this is a casual encounter, you're using a condom, right?) If you find swallowing unpleasant it is absolutely not a requirement. While most men would *like* if women swallowed after oral sex, they would prefer to *get* oral sex. If you can't stomach semen, don't sweat it. Spit.

If he's clean and you've decided whether or not you want to swallow, you can go ahead with our top tips.

It's not all about his dick. It's not. It's not as though the only part of a man's body that is sensitive is the part between his legs. Before getting down to the "main action," take some time to explore the rest of his body with your lips, fingers, and tongue. Try his neck, clavicle, nipples, stomach, and the joint between his leg and torso. Try building up the anticipation a bit and he'll be hot and heavy *well* before you're ready to put anything in your mouth.

Don't forget about your hands. Yes, your mouth is the main star, here, but use your hands to help you out a bit. Hold the base of the penis and stroke it. Also, you can use your hands to keep the action going if you decide you want to pull off his penis for a breath of air or to kiss him.

Use the power of words. While you're coming up for air, talk about how great his dick feels in your mouth and how you love his taste. Remember, guys *love it* when women speak well of their penises. Also, try talking about how good he looks all flushed and aroused.

Take your time. Plenty of women tries to rush oral sex and this just ruins it. Don't just get down and suck him into the back of your throat (well, okay, do that *sometimes*), but instead take your time and stroke him, rub your lips against the head of his penis, etc. Do not look like you're in a rush to finish so you can get to a doctor's appointment or something. Be slow and sensual.

You don't have to deepthroat. Of course, if you can get him all the way into your throat, don't let us stop you. But if you find the idea intimidating, you can certainly replicate the feeling by holding the bottom of his shaft firmly, and then wrap your lips just below the head of his penis. Move your hand and mouth in tandem up and down. This will simulate the feeling of deep throating while having nothing actually in your throat. Of course, if you and your man like it a bit rough there's nothing wrong with gagging, but this can take you out of the moment. If it makes you uncomfortable, don't do it.

Talk about your boundaries. Many women have bad experiences with oral because they don't properly voice (or know) their boundaries. If the thought of your man pushing your head on his dick makes you uncomfortable, *tell him that.* If you don't want to actually deep throat, tell him that. On the other hand, if you don't mind if he pulls your hair a bit, tell him that as well. Once both of you know what you are comfortable with, oral will get a lot better for the both of you.

Try lube. While you might not think of lube as a traditional additive for oral sex, it can go a long way toward preventing mouth dryness. Remember that you will need to use a water-soluble lube since you'll obviously end up consuming some of it. Additionally, if you still have issues with the taste of a penis even after it's been washed, getting flavored lubricant can help make the whole thing go down easier.

Take breaks. Anybody who's ever given their man a blowjob knows that you can end up with neck aches and sore jaws. Don't feel as though you have to suck like a Hoover for 30 straight minutes. Take breaks. Pull away and rub the head of his cock against your lips so you can relax your jaw for a bit. Lick. Play with your tongue on the underside of his cock where there are sensitive bundles of nerves. You can even take a break and switch to vaginal sex for a bit if desired.

Feel free to add a little pain to it. This is definitely something that you should discuss with your man beforehand, but a little bit of pain often heightens pleasure to a certain extent. You could try digging your fingernails in a bit on his hips as you suck, or maybe constricting your mouth hard enough to cause him a bit of pain. *Some* men even enjoy a bit of tooth on their penis, but you should *definitely ask* before trying that.

If he has a foreskin, use it. Not all men do, but if your man is unsnipped, using the foreskin as a way to tease during oral sex is a great way to send him through the roof. Use your tongue to work it down the sides of his shaft as he gets more erect.

Consider temperature play. Popping an ice cube in your mouth can provide a very refreshing sensation. Another thing to try would be sipping a cup of warm tea or coffee. Some men even enjoy the feeling of peppermint or cinnamon red-hots!

Moan. Making noise isn't just for his benefit - though, it definitely will help turn him on a lot! - it's for yours. The more noise that you make while you're going down on your man will help to excite you as well.

Masturbate. Trust us, nothing is going to get your man hotter than having you be so excited that you have to touch yourself while going down on him. (This may actually end the experience earlier than you expect.)

Don't forget his testicles. Again, ask your man before playing too much with them - some men are very sensitive - but testicles have tons of nerve endings in them. For an extra bang, when he's getting ready to orgasm, give his balls a little tug. It will send him over the edge.

Ask him what he likes. Just because you've done oral sex before doesn't mean you know what's good on *all* penises. Ask your man if he has any specific moves that he likes. Some men may like a lot of suction while others prefer a little. Remember, direct communication works wonders with men and is very likely to get you what you want.

Consider the 69. Hey, it's the best of both worlds - he goes down on you while you go down on him. Talk about a distraction!

Chapter 10: How to Spice Things Up In the Sack

It can be easy to fall into the same-old-same-old when it comes to sex with your man, and that's not good for him or you. You can ensure to keep on blowing his mind by keeping things a little more interesting. If you're not sure where to start, we can help you out with that!

Get all dressed up. Nothing like a little bit of clothing fun to make things a bit different. Lingerie is probably the most traditional thing here, but you can always make it a bit more exciting with French maid costumes or the like. Don't forget that he can always get dressed up, too! Maybe he could dress up like a sexy air conditioner repairman. (Just a suggestion.)

Don't look away. The next time you have sex with your man, try keeping your eyes open the entire time. You may not even realize it, but you very likely have a tendency to close your eyes during sex and escape off into your own little world. If you keep your eyes focused on your partner during sex, you may very well be surprised at how intimate the moment can become. (Hey, spicing it up isn't *just* about getting wilder than normal! Getting more emotionally intimate than normal can be extremely powerful!)

Get down with the Kama Sutra. There's a reason why this book has been around for centuries, and it's largely because it has a bunch of amazing sex moves in it. Some of the moves in the Kama Sutra are… astoundingly complex and probably shouldn't be attempted unless you are a gymnast, but there are some that are considerably more doable in nature.

For instance, consider trying **making a fire**, where you rub your husband's erect penis like you're trying to start a fire with a stick. You may also try **spiraling the stalk**, which is where you put one hand on top of another and twist them in opposite directions. **The thousand yonis** is a move where you put one hand on the top of his penis and stroke down, followed immediately by the other hand. Repeat with the first hand over and over. "Yoni" is the Sanskrit word for "vagina," and this move supposedly feels like he's entering a thousand different vaginas!

Again, these don't require an Olympic background in gymnastics to complete and are certainly an interesting twist on the same tired old hand job.

Don't feel as though you have to spend a lot of money to try something new. You may be a bit hesitant to drop a paycheck on a sex toy emporium, but you can definitely get kinky without having to spend a mint. For instance, common items around the house that can be used for a spanking scene involve spatulas, pans, spoons, or ping-pong paddles. You can try using a rolling pin to give massages. Heck, go into your laundry room while your dryer is set to tumble and take a tumble yourself on top of it!

Bring food into it! Food play is simple, sexy, and fun. Try covering your man in chocolate or whipped cream or pudding or anything you'd like to lick and then lick it off of him in lines. You can also feed chocolate-dipped fruit to each other. (The only thing to be careful of is sugary items around your vagina. If sugar gets into your vagina it becomes a prime breeding ground for yeast, which you definitely want to avoid.)

Try some light bondage. There are indeed people out there who are into their chains, but if those are just too intimidating for you, there are other, lighter ways to make it work. Consider using neckties or scarves to tie wrists or ankles together. If you're really nervous, you can just wrap them around your wrists and hold the ends of the ties in your hands. If you want to get into bondage a little more seriously but not spend a lot of money, consider investing in zip ties. They are virtually unbreakable and very inexpensive. (Just make sure to wrap a scarf or sock around body parts first so that the zip tie doesn't accidentally cut too much into the skin.)

Put on a show for your partner. Masturbating in front of your partner isn't just a way to turn him on, but it's also a great way to show him what you do when you're alone. After all, you definitely know what you like, right? Show your partner and you'll reap the benefits! It's also very educational for you as well to watch your man masturbate. And even if you've never thought of that being a sexy thing to watch, you may be surprised. You like to watch your man in pleasure when he's having sex with you, right? It's also fun to watch him in the throes of pleasure when he's going at it solo!

Consider toys. Again, they aren't necessary, but they *can* up your game to a whole other level. You don't need to go with giant rubber penises or massive vibrators, either. There are tons of much more discreet products to choose from if you're a bit hesitant. There is also a wide *array* of products for you to choose from, including things like Ben Wa balls or anal beads or cock rings. The options are literally endless so get on the internet and do some research. If you're not shy, you can go to your local sex shop and see what they have on display.

Share your fantasies with each other. As mentioned earlier in the book, if you feel hesitant to talk about your sexual fantasies with your partner, that's a bad sign. Additionally, just because you *talk* about your fantasies does not mean that you have to actually act them out. (And depending on the fantasy, fulfilling it may not be possible, anyway. Your man may have a thing for 20-armed tentacle monsters, but even if you were down with the same thing it would be rather hard to find a tentacle monster to play with.)

The simple act of sharing may turn you on and get you closer. Not to mention, simply talking about sex may be enough to make you hot.

Talk dirty to him. Most men love phone sex. Even if you're going to see each other later on tonight, there's no reason not to engage in a bit of afternoon delight with him on his lunch break. This will turn him on early in the day and keep you on his mind until he gets home at night. If you can't bring yourself to actually utter the words on the phone (or if you're in an area that is too public for dirty talk), send some sexy texts.

Consider sexy pictures. Many women aren't comfortable with sending nudes to their men, but men definitely love it when women do. So go find a room with favorable lighting and get your selfie on. Another great idea is to have your partner take pictures of you, or perhaps video tape having sex together. Men, in particular are very visual creatures, so having lots of visual stimulation of you on hand is a sure way to get you into his mind. Also considering asking *him* to send *you* some sexy pictures. This isn't as common, but most men are very happy to oblige!

Don't get scripted. Sex is wonderful when it's spontaneous! Make sure that you sometimes jump him when he gets out of the shower or right when he walks in the room. Many people get in the trap of scheduling their sex like it's an errand, rather than a true expression of love and affection. Keep your man guessing, and make it clear that you're open for unexpected advances on his part as well. This will keep your sex life fresh and exciting.

Consider investing in a book collection. Books like this can help you keep things exciting and give you ideas for when you get stuck in a rut. But don't feel as though you have to be consigned solely to advise books! Getting great sexual fantasy literature will give you great ideas as well.

Watch porn together. While many women don't exactly like visual pornography all that much, it's a rare man who does not. Even if you're not that into porn yourself, consider watching it with your man. He will likely find it an unbelievable turn on, and it may be a source of new ideas, just like your book collection is.

Don't get focused on the end goal. Even if you have the most amazing sex life in the world, both partners are not going to orgasm all the time. You may be under stress or your body just isn't feeling it that day for whatever reason. This can also happen with him - he's not a sex machine either. Don't be goal-oriented when it comes to sex; be experience-oriented. You can have an encounter where you, your man, or both you and your man do not orgasm and that doesn't make the sex bad.

Laugh. Sex is funny. You'll make funny noises and occasionally you'll be in the middle of a complicated move when he rolls over onto his car keys, gets poked in the ass, and loses his erection. It happens. Also, make sure to engage in playful acts that may not be directly sex-related. For instance, try buying body paint or playing strip Twister or something like that. This will keep your sex lives more fun, and create that environment of intimacy where both of you will be more inclined to trust and engage with the other.

Chapter 11: Experiment with Anal on Yourself and On Him

Anal sex gets its own chapter since it's such a taboo-yet-often-desired subject. Many people are uncomfortable with anal sex in any fashion whatsoever, and if this is you, there's no reason to feel ashamed about it. If you can't even stomach the thought of something going "up there" or entering your man's back door, that's completely fair.

However, anal sex is as popular as it is for a reason. If it's done correctly it shouldn't be painful. There are tons of nerve endings in the anus. As for your man, he may think that it's "gay," as if gay men somehow have a different physiology than he does. They do not.

Even with a man who may be very hesitant to try anal sex, many who eventually take the plunge wonder why they haven't done so sooner. If you're looking for a way to keep your sex life fresh and exciting, you can't do much better than trying to take it on the other side. Here are our tips.

Do not start off with anal on a one night stand. This is just a bad idea. If this is your first time having anal sex, you need to be doing it with a man that you like and trust enough to do it with. If you do it on a one-off, it is likely going to be a terrible experience.

Consider some self-play beforehand. If you're exploring the idea of anal sex on yourself, there's no reason to take a bit of a plunge before in private. Trim your nails and try inserting a (lubricated!) finger or two into your anus. Remember that your anus is *made* to stretch to a certain extent, so a finger or two will be completely manageable. Keep relaxed.

Another good way to get used to anal play is to try toys. For *him*, there are actually very thin probes that are designed to stimulate the prostate, which can be a great way to get a somewhat-reluctant man to give it a shot. These toys are thin enough to where they won't really stretch the anus but angled to hit your man's inner g-spot, which will result in an incredibly intense orgasm. Other good options include anal beads or butt plugs. Remember that anything going into your anus should have a flared base so it can't get lost inside of you. These toys are great to incorporate into your "regular" sex routine so that everybody can get used to anal play before moving on to the "real deal."

Talk about it with your partner beforehand. Whether you are going to try anal sex on him or on you, you need to ensure that all expectations are laid out on the table as well as boundaries. Neither one of you should want to hurt or freak out the other, so having a conversation about expectations is a must.

Get turned on and relaxed. If you or he like wine, now's not a bad time to have a glass. Also, lots of foreplay is absolutely necessary for successful anal sex. This is an essential step. If you are considering engaging in anal sex and you don't feel like you're about to orgasm on the spot, you probably need more foreplay before you go any further.

Stay hygienic. This is especially important for your vagina, as any cross-contamination between the anus and the vagina may very well result in infection. If you are on the receiving end and he is using his penis, you may want to consider using a condom even if you don't for normal vaginal sex. This way you can just remove the condom after and he doesn't have to take a break to go wash himself. Any toys that are used in the anus should remain anus-only for the most part (though glass, being that it is not porous, can certainly be washed in a dishwasher if you aren't shy about it). If you want to use a dildo that you also use in your vagina, put a condom on it first.

Do not forget the lube! The importance of lubricant during anal sex cannot be overstated. You should use plenty of lubricants and it should be silicone-based - water-based lube can break down faster. Remember that the anus is not a self-lubricating orifice like the vagina is, so all lubrication (and there must be lubrication) needs to be brought in by an outside source.

Remember that the anus is meant to stretch. Many women are afraid of anal sex with a real penis because they believe the experience will be extremely painful, but this is not necessarily the case. The anus is meant to stretch, and most men aren't going to be large enough to stretch it in any unnatural way.

Your first time might not work out so well. Particularly in the event where you are the one of the receiving end and your man is using his penis to penetrate you… he's probably pretty excited. Most men dream of anal sex but not all of them get it. Particularly if it is also *his* first time doing this, the experience… may end a bit prematurely. Plus, you may need to keep reminding him to take it slow. Most men only encounter anal sex through porn videos, which feature literal pros and are not good instructional manuals.

You may experience some cramping and cleanup afterward. Particularly in the event that you have anal sex without a condom on you and he orgasms inside of you… any lube or semen that was expelled into you will need to come back out. You may want to be in private for this part, as it can be a bit messy. Additionally, for the first couple of times you have anal sex you may experience mild cramping in your abdomen. This is normal.

Many men and women grow to *love* anal sex, due to the high amount of nerve endings that the anus has (more than in the vagina!). With enough experimentation and trust, this can definitely knock your sex life up to the next level and beyond.

Chapter 12: Consider "Guest Stars"

Many men fantasize about threesomes. For some, they're considered to be the holy grail of sex. However, they can also cause massive amounts of problems - probably everybody has some kind of a drama-mama story about a threesome gone wrong and somebody getting kicked out of the house over it.

While threesomes can be fun and kinky, they also need to be handled with care. We've got some tips for how to make your sexual threesomes work for you.

Don't pick a friend. Don't pick a friend. *Don't pick a friend.* There. We've said it three times. Picking a friend for a threesome is just going to result in a mess. Plus, it can be kind of awkward to ask your childhood best friend if she'd like to bump uglies with you and your man. Just don't do it. It is highly likely the friend will say no, anyway, and that'll be the weird elephant in the corner of the room for the rest of your relationship. Your friend probably thinks of either you or your man like family, anyway, not a potential hookup. The only exception is if the friend has secretly been lusting over you or your man for a while, and this carries problems of its own.

Speaking of "problems," no romantic feelings. If there is *any chance whatsoever* of romantic feelings between your threesome partner, your man, or you, you should absolutely not pick that person. Things will just get messy. Absolutely positively no exes! That is simply going to end in disaster.

You may want to try going with an easygoing stranger. There's a reason why online dating exists these days. Sites like Tinder and OKCupid make it easy to surf and try to find somebody that seems all right that neither one of you know. This will also make it easy to either set up a sex-only situation with that person if they want to come back multiple times. A one-and-done works well in this situation as well. Again, you don't want to end up with a crazy person, but you also absolutely do not want somebody that you know, frankly. A good bet is trying to get somebody through an online dating site, and then taking him or her out to dinner or something beforehand. Treat it like a cross between a get-to-know-you and a job interview.

Use protection. Protection is an absolute must for all parties during threesomes. Condoms, dental dams, the whole nine yards. This goes doubly so if you are getting down with somebody you don't know well at all. Unless your Tinder hook up comes along with a clean STD sheet, put barriers between them and your partner. Generally speaking, it's best practice for you and your man to use protection with each other too during a threesome, just to ensure that all of the bases are covered.

Make sure that you are paying attention to your partner. It can be exciting to be caught up in something new, but you need to ensure that you are paying enough attention to your man. *Also*, you will want to speak to him beforehand and ensure that he knows to pay enough attention to *you*. It's possible that your man will get wrapped up in the excitement of somebody shiny and new, and this can make you feel neglected. In the event that this starts to occur, try not to take it personally - it may help if you have some sort of secret signal to let him know that you are feeling ignored.

Keep involved. Even if you aren't directly taking place in whatever is going on at the moment (let's say your man and the other partner are kissing), try stroking a hand down their backs or gently tugging hair. Don't get into a position where you look like you are sulking in a corner. If you don't know what to do, simply touch the other two people.

If one partner leaves the room for whatever reason, the action should stop. If your need to go to the toilet, your man and the third person should take a short break as well. This will help you and your man feel as though you are a team in the threesome. Remember, you and your man are coming into this as an item - you should act like it.

Talk about what is and is not okay to do with the third party beforehand. Is it okay to kiss the third party? Penetrate? Discuss with your man what your go-aheads and no-ways are when it comes to the third person involved in your tryst. Once you have this hammered out between you, make sure that this is communicated to the third person. You don't want to have your man agree not to kiss the other woman, but then have the other woman lunge forward and take his mouth!

Don't leave hickies. This is just good general practice. If your man leaves hickies on the third party, you're likely to be upset. If the third party leaves hickies on your man… do you want to be looking at that for the next week? It's just better off to avoid love bites altogether during a threesome.

Try to orgasm around the same time. If one person orgasms well before the others, that first person may indeed start to lose interest in the threesome before the other two do, and this can create issues. Try to ensure that the orgasms happen in a timely manner. Obviously, this can cause some timing challenges, as it's unlikely you're going to be able to make everybody come at *exactly* the same time, but it's helpful if you can at least ensure it's within 5 minutes of each other. Typically speaking, it's a better idea to focus on the orgasms of the women first, since men have an easier time with this.

Try to orgasm with your partner. Ideally, the partner that is the same sex as the third member should orgasm with the partner. So if the partner is a woman, your man should orgasm with you, not the third woman. If the partner is male, you should orgasm with your man, not with the third man. This helps reinforce the primary importance of the relationship between you and your man.

The other person really shouldn't sleep over if at all possible. Granted, if you have an established threesome relationship already this may be less of an issue, but the third person should never seem as though they are getting between you and your man. In the event that your third person is in a situation where they can't get home after the

threesome (say that the public transportation has stopped),
it's better if they sleep on the downstairs couch or in a guest
room as compared to in the bed with you and your man.

Talk about it with your partner after, and be honest.
Was there any point where you felt jealous? Where he felt
left out? How did the encounter leave you both feeling after
the threesome?

Threesomes are a very powerful way to bring some spice
into your relationship, but they have to be handled very
carefully. If you and your man don't communicate well, then
you shouldn't even attempt this.

Chapter 13: Try Different Kinds of Kink

This is somewhat related to "spicing it up," but this is a list of suggestions for people who are really ready to get out of their comfort zone and get their kink on. If you're looking for some ways to wild it up a bit, give these suggestions a shot.

Consider going to a "munch." If you've tried threesomes and they aren't enough for you anymore, you can definitely get wilder. There are groups you can join where people who are into BDSM or other scenes can chat. Often, these start off at a "munch," which is a non-sexual gathering of people who are potentially interested in alternative sexual scenes. These gatherings are usually very comfortable (nobody is going to be dressed in fetish gear), and designed as a meet-and-greet.

This is a great way for you and your man to consider getting into the alternative scene if you are interested. There are munches in cities across the world - if you seek, ye shall find.

Consider getting involved in virtual fetish sites. If you are intrigued by the idea of alternative sexuality but either doesn't live in an area where you can attend a munch or are simply too shy, consider checking out a website like fetlife.com. Here, behind the safety of your computer screens, you and your man can explore more fetishes and wild things than you ever thought could exist.

Consider going to a sex club. Depending on where you are, you may very well have actual sex clubs in your area. Some of these are BDSM dungeons where you can go to watch others play or give it a try yourself. If you're curious, this is a great way to explore the more exhibitionist part of fetish culture. And, who knows, one day it might be you and your man on the stage engaging in some sweaty fetish fun?

Don't forget about pornography. If you're curious about certain kinks, feel free to watch some videos on the subject to see if it's something that actually turns you on or not. It very well may not. Or you might discover a pleasure you never knew existed. Steamy erotica is a good choice for this as well.

Just give it a shot! Hey, if you want to try it, try it. If you want to try watersports, get in the shower and have at it. If you want to dress your man up like a girl and put makeup on him, give it a shot if he's willing. There's nothing wrong with giving anything you'd like to try a go. It will help you open up your sex life further and ensure that things in the sack don't ever get boring!

Conclusion

Thank for making it through to the end of this book, let's hope it was informative and able to provide you with all of the tools you need to achieve your goals whatever they may be. We've enjoyed talking with you about your man and hope that you'll find this information useful in your endeavors!

The next step is to get out there and start communicating with your man! Start talking about your hopes and dreams, and do everything you need to do in order to connect with him on an emotional, physical, and mental level. If you take the advice in this ebook and apply it to your romantic and sexual life, you will have no problem blowing your man's mind and having the sex you've always dreamed of, no matter what it is. Whether you want to make sweet love or get down in a fetish dungeon, you deserve to create the sex life you want with a man who adores you. You've got this!

There are millions of men out there, so get out there and make them all fall head over heels. You may be surprised at how easy getting that man to fall in love with you actually is once you apply our tool set correctly. Not only will this advice ensure that you have a great sex life, but you will have better relationships overall and enjoy the company of your man much more if you understand him better. We hoped this book has helped you do that!

Introduction Book 3

The following chapters will cover many different aspects of women's sexuality, and things that a woman, or man, can do to improve the woman's sex life. The world of sex, especially women's sexuality, has changed a lot for the past several centuries. Things that are used to be forbidden are happening, things that used to happen are now forbidden. With all these changes, there's no wonder that women have a hard time expressing their sexual desires. This book is here to help a woman work past those hindarnces and open up a sexual lifestyle they have always wanted. Don't think that the info is only for women, though. Men can also learn a thing or two from this book to help their ladies open up their sex life.

Chapter 1: A Brief History of Women's Sexuality

The female sexuality has changed remarkably over several centuries, from the vast amount of customs found during the early colonial days to the 19th-century repression, and the 20th-century liberalization of behavior and attitudes. A lot of the changes have happened to women with the use of cultural training, medical influences, and the interpretation and expectation of men. There are some female sexual behaviors that were started by the women themselves by acting in what they thought was the best for them considering what they have available at the time. This is true, especially, of the 19th century.

Historical Sex Beliefs

In the Chinese, Japanese, and Indian ancient civilizations, female sexuality was handled through several commentaries and writings. The *Kama Sutra* is an ancient Indian text that talks about sexuality and sex and looks at female in the context of their sexual pleasure and sexuality.

One psychoanalytical text explains that the Madonna-whore complex happens when a man desires sexual experiences with women he views as degraded, but he is unable to desire a respectable woman sexually. Sigmund Freud was the first person to describe this.

Throughout the history, many cultures have seen female sexuality as being secondary to that of male, and as needing to be controlled with the use of restrictions. Traditional practices, like enforced chastity and modesty, have worked to place restrictions mainly on women, without enforcing the same kind of restrictions on men.

Controversial practices, like female genital mutilation (FGM), have been seen as a way to try and nullify a woman's sexuality completely. FGM is still a common practice in some areas of the Middle East and Africa, and some immigrant communities within some Western countries even though it is outlawed. The procedure normally happens to a young girl before she turns 15.

Other methods that some cultures use to control female behavior and sexuality include the threat of death such as honor killings. These killings have been justified through things like refusing to take part in an arranged marriage, being a part of a relationship that their relatives disapprove of, having sexual relations outside of their marriage, being a rape victim, or wearing clothing that is seen as inappropriate.

A chastity belt is another historical device that was used to control a female's sexual behavior. It is an item of clothing that is locked on to prevent the woman from having sex. Women wore these belts to protect their chastity, which prevented masturbation as well as sexual access.

Before the Europeans colonized the US, Native Americans viewed female sexuality with an open mind, particularly for the younger and unmarried women. However, when the Europeans arrived, they imposed more rigid views. These restrictions were particularly harsh for women in the Puritan colonies.

Medieval Times

Contrary to what medieval romance novels may tell you, the scientific theory of sexual reproduction in medieval times had a big emphasis on the woman's orgasm. They believed that it was required if their act of sex was going to make a baby. To give you an idea of the important, it shows up in many medieval texts, starting in the 13th century.

In theory, this may seem like good news for the women of the 13th century, but it actually wasn't. They based their beliefs on the idea that a woman's sexual organs were the inverted version of a man's, which meant that a woman ejaculated in some fashion, which is why they believed a female orgasm was a requirement.

The biggest problem with this belief is that it is still being used today by "legitimate rape" apologists such as Todd Akin, who believe that the pleasure of a woman is needed to conceive, which, in their eyes, means that if one was raped and ended up pregnant, it wasn't actually "rape" in its context if the woman has had orgasm during the process.

Victorian-Era

When you think of the Victorian-era sex, what comes to mind? Marriages of social bartering and convenience? Corsets? Lots of repressions?

Actually, the way people tend to view this time in sexual history could be more than a little warped. To really understand what the women of the time were like we should look at Clelia Duel Mosher's MD work. Long before Alfred Kinsey came to be, Dr. Mosher was looking into the sexual tendencies of the Victorian women.

She started her work in the 1890s, and it spanned over two decades. During this time, she spoke with 45 women about their sexual preferences and habits, from how frequently they experienced an orgasm to if they ever lusted after somebody that wasn't their spouse.

Unfortunately, Dr. Mosher's report was published during her life. Carl Degler, a historian, professor, and author, is the reason why we know her report. He found her papers in 1973 in the Stanford University archives and published his own analysis the next year.

In her report, she found that not having an orgasm sucked, even back then. Some of her respondents mentioned that a lack of climax was "bad, even disastrous," and they even continue saying she went through "nerve-wracking-unbalancing if such conditions continue for any length of time."

One woman had more to say about the orgasm gap in the 19th century that men hadn't been trained properly in this area of their sex life. It looks as if women have been taking their sexual pleasure very seriously for several centuries, even if the majority of the culture hasn't.

They didn't have sex just for procreation. One woman kept up the Victorian stereotype by saying, "I cannot recognize as true marriage that relation unaccompanied by a strong desire for children," she even went so far to say that a married couple that had sex only for pleasure was nothing more than "legalized prostitution." But there were many other women that disagreed with this view.

There was one woman that believed pleasure was a good enough reason for sex, while another woman said that babies didn't have anything to do with sex: "Even a slight risk of pregnancy, and then we deny ourselves the intercourse, feeling all the time that we are losing that which keeps us closest to each other."

Dr. Mosher's findings are more than just another history lesson. In Degler's analysis, he wrote that in the Victorian-era there was some effort to deny women her sexual feelings and to deny them a legitimate expression. The group of women that participated in the survey was not sexless or hostile to their sexual feelings. None of them allowed societal restraints or expectations to stop them from experiencing their feelings and acting on them.

What you can learn the most from Dr. Mosher's work is that no matter what shame you may feel about your sexuality, or whatever pressure you may experience, you're completely normal and you are not alone. So, don't hide it. After all, you may just be the one that ends up proving people wrong a few hundred years down the line.

Another famous belief in the Victorian-era concerning female orgasm is that sexual tension for women was seen as a "wandering womb" or "hysteria."

Having it be believed that an orgasm was a medical necessity to keep your womb from driving you crazy, orgasm as pathology basically, isn't fun or very helpful to the idea that a partner and husband may want to provide this pleasure.

Sex in Religions

When it comes to sex in religious text, most of them have the same thing to say about it. Abdessamad Dialmy states that the Islamic views of sex are paradoxical because they allow and encourage sex, but only if it is between heterosexual and married couples. Even still they have a discriminatory view of female and male sexuality since they view sex as a male-centered act; he is on top, he should dominate, and he should have multiple wives and concubines. While the Sunna and Quran both encourage female climax, it has nothing to do with their pleasure, but it is seen as a way of discouraging her from looking for sexual pleasure from other sources.

In most all religions, sex is frowned upon if it happens before a couple is married. Sex isn't supposed to be an act of pleasure; instead, it should be holy and sacred and aimed to create tranquility, love, and affection between spouses.

1900s

In the 1940s, scientist Alfred Kinsey's sex survey provided lots of new information around the orgasm and other sexual behaviors. His survey was very thorough, and he discovered some things that still influence the way people view the female orgasm and to achieve them today.

His Kinsey Report was a huge hit, reported that 40% of the women that took part achieved their first orgasm through masturbation, 5% from "wet dreams," 14% experienced multiple orgasms, and that the women's orgasmic abilities continue to rise until they begin to taper off around 55-60 years of age.

His frankness of the sexual experience, differences between people, and the range of possibilities made the female orgasm a little less elusive and more of a fact.

Now that people believed that the female orgasm existed, arguments start to pop about what it was for.

In Desmond Morris' 1967 book, *The Naked Ape*, he argued that a woman's orgasm could have developed as a way for males to prove they have tenderness, gentleness, determination, and other such qualities needed to bring one about. These were good factors in a man being a good father figure. He also mentions that it could increase the chance of conception by "knocking the woman out" and keeping her in a horizontal position so that the sperm would be able to reach the egg easier, which is utter nonsense.

There were other scientists that came up with a variety of other hypotheses. They included; that a female orgasm didn't have to do with monogamy, but was a way to bond with multiple sex partners; that it helps with fertility by "sucking" up the sperm with vaginal spasms; and that orgasm will increase a woman's likelihood of having more sex, thus giving the species a good chance of survival. Nobody has ever actually come up with a definitive explanation.

The scientific team of Masters and Johnson, who are now the subject of the show *Masters of Sex*, were silently studying sex throughout the 60s that helped to prove that multiple orgasms were real and that a woman could experience an orgasm from clitoral or vaginal stimulation.

Starting in the 70s and 80s, the long-held traditional Western views on female sexuality start to be reassessed and challenged with the start of the sexual revolution. Feminist writers and people who were a part of the feminist movement addressed female sexuality from a woman's perspective instead of allowing the female sexuality to be defined by the male sexuality. Nancy Friday's book *My Secret Garden* was one of the first popular nonfiction books about female sexuality.

Female bisexuality and lesbianism started to emerge as a new topic of interest. The attitudes of feminist towards female sexuality have varied widely throughout the movement. For modern feminism, they advocate for women to have equal access to sexual education and healthcare, and they also agree on the importance of having freedom over their reproductive health, especially when it comes to family planning and birth control. Consent and bodily autonomy are also important concepts in modern views of female sexuality.

The 2000s and Beyond

Now that the orgasm has established itself as part of the female sexuality was beginning to gain traction. Scientists began to line up to prove the benefits of it: if they couldn't find a reproductive or sexual function, it had to have some fun stuff, right?

Female orgasms, amongst many other things, have been discovered to help with pain, boost white blood cells and immune systems, improve brain function, regulate menstruation, and improve emotional and mood closeness.

This should be a good enough reason have one every day, just like vitamins. Not that you can see the ups and downs of female sexuality throughout the years, you can kind of understand why women have such a hard time embracing their sexuality. You never know how the next person is going to view female sexuality, and all this stress is only making things worse. So, let's look at the different things you can do to release your sexuality and not worry about all the beliefs that may have been taught to you over the years.

Chapter 2: Understanding What a Woman Wants

Feminine women work on a whole different level than masculine men. The masculine brain relies on its ability to make things happen so that they experience certainty. The feminine brain relies on the use of communication so that they experience certainty.

This may seem like a minute difference, but that small difference in the most fundamental and basic way you engage in life has huge ramifications for your entire life.

Let's look at a few things that a woman will do that seems pointless and foreign to many guys, but makes perfect sense to the woman. Keep in mind; these examples are looking at the two extremes of a spectrum. There aren't that many people out there that are always feminine or always masculine. A person's attitude will fluctuate through the hour, day, week, month, and even each minute. But each person has their own "natural essence" that their default personality is.

The Indecisive Woman

To most men, a woman will seem indecisive. But they aren't indecisive; their mind works in a different way. When it comes to a man, making a decision and performing a job will allow them to experience certainty. When it comes to a woman, making sure that everybody is on the same page and approves of the decision gives them certainty.

It's not that they are indecisive; they just don't actually care about the decisions that are made. They don't base their certainty on what decision is made and what could come from the decision. They base their certainty on how people view their decision. They care about making sure everybody is being looked after and that they are happy than actually getting a job done. Trying to get a woman to be decisive is just like trying to get a man to have a conversation without coming to a certain conclusion.

Women and Their Phone

With a man, reaching to a conclusion, whether they do it through finishing a job or coming up with a decision gives them the chance to experience more certainty. This means for a man, he gets on the phone, discusses something, comes to a conclusion, and then ends the call.

For women, communicating and connecting with others give them more certainty. This is why women like to talk on the phone and connect, cry, laugh, and talk regardless of the subject they are talking about.

This may seem pointless, frustrating, and confusing for the men, it is the best way for women to feel good and experience certainty.

Women and Their Clothes

For most men, the clothes they own is picked based on its ability to help them with a task. This could mean being comfortable, working out, or finishing job. This is because it gives them the ability to feel certain.

For a woman, clothes have a different role. Since their certainty is based on communication, and the way a person dresses affects their communication, then clothing plays a part in how certain they feel.

Having the right shoes to make your favorite dress is important. This may seem like a ridiculous idea for men, because the shoes aren't going to help complete a task, having the best articles of clothing for a woman is important. Although in the present days, men also start to dress according to how they feel. It is slightly different in the context of women but the same reason for their choice of clothes can be observed.

Women and Sensitivity

Men's certainty is based on their ability to do something that makes a difference. This means if they can't achieve their goal of taking action and having something turn out the way they want, they will feel depressed and frustrated.

Women don't respond to not being about taking action unlike men because they don't base their certainty on it. They base their certainty on communication which they become depressed, disappointed, and frustrated based on their communication. This is why they tend to be more sensitive to communication because it is how they achieve their emotional basis.

If you tell a woman that she looks horrible in a pair of pants is just like keeping a man from being able to make a house that he needs to have in order to stay dry and warm.

10 Important Things about a Woman's Brain

1. *As her cycle changes, so does she*

80% of women are affected by PMS, but in fact, a woman is affected by her cycle every single day of the month. Hormones levels are constantly fluctuating in her body and brain, which changed her outlook, sensitivity, and energy.

Around ten days after menstruation has started, just before she ovulates, women will often feel sassier. They will unconsciously dress sexier as they experience surges of testosterone and estrogen prompts them to start looking for sexual partners in their fertile phase.

In another week their progesterone rises, which makes women want to cuddle up with a book with a cup of tea. The next week, when they go through progesterone withdrawal, they start to feel irritated or weepy. For many women, their mood is at its worst 12-24 hours before their period begins. They don't really have any free will over this.

2. *She is intuitive*

Men will sometimes feel as if women are psychics or mind readers, but this intuitive ability is more biological. During evolution, women were likely chosen based on their ability to keep children alive, which involves figuring out what a child needs. This is one of the main reasons why women tend to score higher on reading nonverbal cues.

They are better at remembering other's physical appearances, and they can correctly identify body language based on tones of voice, postures, and facial expressions. This isn't a skill that is only limited to child rearing.

3. *She stays away from aggression*

Stressful situations cause the "fight or flight" response in men, but for women, they tend to try to "tend or befriend." This means that instead of a physical response, they will try to form a strategic, sometimes manipulative, alliance. Through evolution, women have moved past physical aggression because their children's survival depends more on them.

4. *Her response to anxiety and pain is different*

A woman's brain does not only respond more to stress, but it is less able to handle high-stress levels. The sensitivity to stress has some benefits as well; it will shift a person's mental state from a narrow focus to being more open and flexible. If the anxiety lasts too long, it can cause some problems. This is likely why a woman I more prone to depression, PTSD, and anxiety disorders.

5. *She dislikes conflict but hates a lack of response more*

Women have evolved to have more sensitivity to nonverbal cues to stay away from conflict, a state that is intolerable to most women. The chemicals that flood a woman's brain during a conflict, especially in a relationship, is similar to that of a seizure. More than likely due to their ability of "mind reading," women will find a blank expression, or no response, as unbearable. A little girl will work hard to try to get a mime to respond, while a little boy wouldn't feel that determined. A lot of the times, a negative response, to a woman, is better than not getting a response.

6. *She can be easily turned off*

There are certain areas of a woman's brain that has to shut off in order for her to get in the mood, and especially to have an orgasm. There are lots of things that could turn these areas back on.

Women could refuse a man because they feel distrustful, angry, or even because she has cold feet. Menopause, pregnancy, and caring for children also tend to take a toll on her sex drive. If a man wants to make sure they turn-on their woman, they need to plan ahead.

7. *Pregnancy affects her brain*

There is a huge increase in progesterone during the first eight weeks of pregnancy. This causes a woman to feel more sedated. The brain will also shrink during pregnancy, decreasing by about 4% by the time of delivery. Some believe pregnancy hormones cause memory problems, while others believe these changes are to help the brain circuits prepare for motherhood.

8. *Mommy brain affects a woman*

There are monumental changes that a woman experiences after giving birth both socially, emotionally, hormonally, and physically. During evolution, it was uncommon for a woman to be a full-time mother because kin-folk were there to help with rearing the children. The mother's ability to respond adequately to her child impacts the child's development and temperament. Mother Nature has tried to help through breastfeeding. Nursing can help some women work through stress; although too much stress can affect lactation.

9. *Women experience adolescence*

Nobody enjoyed going through the adolescence, the physical and hormonal changes not only caused mood swings and bodily discomfort, but questions of self-identity popped up as well. But, luckily for women, they will go through a second adolescence referred to as perimenopause during their 40s. It will begin around 43 and then reaches its peak at 47 or 48. But of course, this age range is variable among women. With the night sweats and erratic periods, this transition can cause a woman to become a moody teenager again. This will last anywhere between two to nine years, with most being through it by age 52.

10. During their mature years, women love risk

After women have gone through the change, the body hits the advanced stage and gets a second wind. Men, as they get older, has an increased interest in relationships, a mature woman will be drawn to risk conflict, especially if she is an empty nester. She will likely still feel motivated to help other people, but the focus may change from family to global and local communities. She may also want to do things more for herself, and career after years of taking care of others.

Work through Five Mental Blocks

Let's look at the five most common mental blocks women will experience when it comes to expressing her sexuality, and how to work through them.

1. She's afraid she is being judged

This is a fear that tends to hold people back in all areas of their life. This becomes exacerbated because you don't know how another person really has sex, or what they think about. So, it's easy to jump to the conclusion that you're not normal.

Try this: Start by picturing how it would be if you weren't afraid of judgment. Write down the things that you would do and how you would feel if followed your sexuality. Sometimes all you need to do is tell your partner you want to ask for more sexually, but you're afraid of what they will think. See how they react. If you are with the right person, showing some vulnerability can create an authentic relationship and make for better sex.

2. She's insecure

Insecurity can show up in many ways, such as worrying your partner won't be happy, or you don't deserve the desire. You could be afraid that you can't please your partner, and you may even think you will drive them away.

Try this: Decide if your insecurity is personal, or part of your relationship. If it's personal insecurity, you have to work hard to make sure you don't project it onto your partner. If it's based on your relationship, think of the possibilities. Is there an actual threat? Do you ever think about cheating on them? Are the two of you out of sync? Maybe the relationship just needs a tune-up, or you just need a little more affirmation from your partner.

3. *She's unsure of what she wants*

A lot of women aren't even sure of the sexual options they have. You can't make a request if you don't know what you can choose from.

Try this: Try watching some racy movies or reading erotica. Talk with friends you can trust and find out what they like. Visit a workshop at a local female owned and operated sex shop. The main thing is to explore the different possibilities.

4. *She's afraid of rejection*

One of the main reasons why a person will avoid expressing what they desire is because they are afraid of hearing no. You could end up projecting this fear onto your partner.

Try this: Quit taking no personally. There are a lot of different reasons why a person could tell you no, and they have nothing to do with yours. No is most of the time a self-care response. It works as a boundary that the person needs. It will take time to master the skill of not feeling hurt when you hear the word no.

5.   She does what she thinks she is supposed to

Society has a limited view of sex and pleasure. The main idea of sex, especially for heterosexuals, is the main thing despite the fact that women need the foreplay for pleasure and sex ends once the man ejaculates. This is what is learned during sex ed. This means that most women are conditioned to strive for a vaginal orgasm which most women are unable to achieve.

Try this: Talk truthfully to your partner about trying sex that isn't just focused solely on intercourse. This could open the door for both of you to begin thinking more creatively. You two could come up with a whole menu of sexual options.

Chapter 3: Boost Your Self-Esteem

If you were to look into your partner's eyes, what are you going to see? Hopefully, you would see support, love, and respect. Now, do you think that you deserve those feelings? This answer is important because how you feel about yourself will play an important part in your chances of maintaining a close relationship and enjoying your sexual relationship.

Self-esteem is how you view yourself with how you cope with all of the basic parts of life, and whether or not you believe you deserve happiness. If you don't believe that you deserve happiness, you may end up believing that you're not worthy of sensual, full, rich, and sexual life.

There is even sexual self-esteem, which is defined as how you see yourself as a sexual person. Do you view yourself as appealing? Competent in a sexual sense? How do you view yourself when you are with someone else? These are all important parts of your sexual self-esteem.

Ideally, you should have high sexual self-esteem. But if you have ever experienced emotional or physical abuse, been sexually embarrassed, harassed, or insulted, then it's likely that your sexual self-esteem has suffered. The damage from these types of negative situation can be so great, even if they were called sexually demeaning names, that one person has even said that a damaged sexual self-esteem is a disability that can interfere with functioning.

Women who suffer from low sexual self-esteem will often have problems with sex and is more likely to be involved in higher risk sexual behaviors, like multiple unprotected sex partners.

Even if you have never experienced abuse, you could still have low self-esteem for reasons like being middle-aged or older in a world that puts more value on being beautiful and youthful or being adventurous in a sexual sense.

To take this another step further, think about how you view yourself as a sexually attractive person. This has a lot to do with how you view your body, especially your weight. A study performed at Duke University discovered that women who were overweight didn't want people to see them undressed, had a low sexual desire, avoided sexual encounters, had problems with performance, and didn't enjoy sex.

The issue with self-esteem can go in the other direction as well; researchers found that women that suffered from sexual dysfunction also have a lack of sexual desire and low self-esteem. The lower their self-esteem was, the less likely they would go get help.

So, let's make a pact to improve your sexual self-esteem. To help you do just that, here are ten things you can do to improve your sexual self-esteem.

1. *Find your inner diva*
Beyoncé has famously stated that when she performs she taps into her alter ego, Sasha Fierce. When this type of persona gives Beyoncé confidence, you can use the same thing to give yourself a confidence boost in the bedroom. Start acting as if you are someone else with attributes to help you feel more confident. The action is preceded by motivation.

2. Look at the bodies of real women

The women we see in TV, movies, and magazines aren't realistic representations. If all you are seeing are size two women and you're a size 12, and then will probably start to feel down. So, you need to take a media break. Go someplace like the gym or somewhere there is a communal dressing room and take notice of how real women actually look. Don't start at them, just notice. This will remind you that sexy comes in all sizes

3. Look at how strong your body is

When you feel completely unsexy, try doing this: view your body as an instrument instead of an ornament. Think of things that remind you of your strength, such as dancing, climbing, running, or childbirth.

4. Play some music

Bypass the alcohol and use music to get in a sexy mood. Sexy music can easily influence the way you view yourself.

5. Stay away from Facebook for a bit

You could blame Facebook for insecurity that you may experience in the bedroom. One Canadian study found that the more often people were on social media, the more they jealous they became of their romantic partners.

6. Speak up about what you want

If you find you have a hard time asking for something in bed, try asking specifically and firmly for things that you want during the day. You can do this by becoming comfortable with asking for certain things at the dry cleaners, restaurants, or at your child's school. As you become more comfortable with your needs and articulating them, soon you will be able to do so with your partner.

7.   Don't watch as many romantic comedies

Everybody loves a good chick flick, but those happy endings could be bringing you down. Research has found a correlation between rom-com movies and relationship dissatisfaction. They cause you to have an unrealistic view of how relationships work.

8.   Get a dimmer switch

Dimming the lights is a quick way to put yourself in the mood. You can also use candlelight if you don't want to invest in a dimmer switch. See how this affects your confidence.

9.   Quit watching the clock

Quit worrying about how long sex should last. If you have watched a love scene in a movie recently then it's not hard to think that great sex has to last for hours. And then when your actual encounter lasts six minutes, you can easily assume something is wrong. In fact, a study performed in 2008 found that sex that was classified as "normal and good" only lasted between three to 13 minutes.

10. Purchase some lingerie

An easy way to improve your self-esteem is with some flattering lingerie. This is especially true if you have suffered from weight fluctuations. Buy something that fits you comfortably now and don't try to wear something that is uncomfortable.

Chapter 4: Improving Intimacy

People often express their desire to love and be loved, to be accepted and known for who we are, to be in a safe relationship, hoping to share out failings and dreams. Is it intimacy that people truly want?

There are so many times when people will use the term intimate in a completely physical context. People can call a couple intimate to express the fact that they have a sexual relationship. But the truth is that this is a narrow and misleading use of the word because there are different types of intimacy:

- Emotional
- Sexual
- Experiential
- Intellectual

Sexual Intimacy

There are times when everybody hungers for a sexual connection, and this is a physical longing. We may not only yearn for intercourse, but also just the presence and touch of another person with their own sensual splendor; the textures, sounds, scents, tastes, and the visual aspects also play a part.

During sex, barriers are lowered, and another person is allowed to your private personal space. This type of intimacy involves some trust and vulnerability. There will be times when everybody wants sex and not lovemaking. This can happen without any attachments, with a bit of affection, or between friends. If you pay attention, you can understand the little nuances of sharing your body and not your heart.

Emotional Intimacy

Sometimes we are interested in finding an emotional connection; accepting yourself, loving yourself, sharing happiness and tough times. People crave comfort, closeness, and trust. People want to have a special connection with a person on a deep emotional level.

This type of intimacy doesn't need physical affection, though for some it can be enhanced by holding hands or a kiss on the cheek.

Two people can be married for years, and they never reach emotional intimacy; remember that intimacy is not a destination but an experience or a group of feelings. Communication is important when it comes to emotional intimacy, but people tend to communicate about life superficially.

People also use activities, humor, and sarcasm to fill up the time they spend together. Whether intentional or not, people tend to "deflect and protect" so that they can avoid transparency and vulnerability that people need in order to thrive as a couple.

The vulnerability that is needed for emotional intimacy produces anxiety for many people. A good way to help get rid of this anxiety is to allow plenty of time to pass so that you can establish trust. The vulnerability can still prove to be tough especially if you're out of practice.

While many people view sex as relationship glue from where intimacy and communication will flow, others see emotional intimacy as a prerequisite to a good sex life. So, what if this vulnerability isn't going to happen? What if your significant other isn't willing, or can't communicate on a deep and personal way? Even if you have amazing sex, will an unsatisfying amount of emotional intimacy leave you wanting more?

Everybody Experiences Intimacy Differently

Sexual and emotional intimacy tends to be tricky because there are no absolutes. What everybody needs when it comes to intimacy can vary. The way one person deeply shares will be different than the next.

In the same way, our comfort with emotional and sexual intimacy is going to change some over time and evolve with the relationship we're in and the circumstances. Take this, for example, a woman who was married for 20 years is now divorced. To say the very least, the mere thought of stripping off in front of a new lover may cause anxiety, so she could choose to establish a mutual emotional intimacy foundation before any sexual activity. Or she could go the route of detachment with a hookup instead of putting her heart out there.

There are some people that are found with keeping sex at arm's length from their emotions, which makes their lives a lot less complicated. There are single mothers out there that explicitly operate like this, given that having to deal with their ex, raising their kids, and hold down a job is an emotional overload.

There are others that need a convergence of sexuality with connection, agreement, transparency, and trust, which is the definition of emotional intimacy. This all depends on communication and time.

But passion isn't decided through emotional intimacy, just like emotional intimacy doesn't have to have any physical contact. Love is able to happen at an emotional remove or even a sexual remove for that matter. Connection, sex, love: these are what make up the best mix of satisfaction and comfortableness for both people in a relationship.

How to Deepen Your Sexual Connection

If you're interested in bringing more intimacy into your sex life with your partner, instead of it just being sex, here are five things that can help deepen that intimacy.

1. *Realize the importance of creating an intimate friendship with your significant other*

A lot of people tend to focus too much on the technique during sex. However, your relationship with your partner is a lot more important for feelings of intimacy. The sense of safety, mutual trust, and emotional connection in your relationship is needed in order to bring the intimacy to your sexual desires. Basically, you should work up to the feeling that you are living with somebody that you crave so much, that makes the actual sex even more pleasurable.

2. *Become deeply connected with your body*

All the stresses of every day like can keep many of us from being able to keep a thorough and consistent self-care routine. As a result, many will devote only a small amount of time enjoying, embracing, and exploring our own bodies. The effects of stress will often trickle into the sex life. When a person doesn't have an intimate and comfortable relationship with their self, it's almost impossible to create an intimate and comfortable sexual relationship with their partner. If you make a space to love, feel, and explore your own body, you will be able to communicate better about what you want, what makes you feel fulfilled, and what you crave.

3. *Speak up*

A big reason as to why sex will begin to feel like a routine, and a lot less passionate, is because there isn't enough communication. You may see it as overreacting if you voice how upset you were when your partner gave your friend flirty eyes. It would seem unnecessary to speak about how upset you were when you partner didn't ask your opinion when planning your date. But look at it this way: when you suppress your emotion, it isn't going to go away, it will show up again somewhere else.

A way that it will show up is through suppressed intimacy, any form of intimacy. If you can shorten the time between when you were upset about letting that person know, the lower your resentment levels will be. Less negativity means you will have a better willingness to receive and give in different ways, especially with sex.

4. *Embrace the dark, light, and everything in between*

It's easy for couples to fall into sexual monotony, and it typically coexists with safety. But if you can widen your expressiveness range, it can open the door to a deeper spiritual connection, and this typically means getting out of your safety zone. You may be worried about bringing up something that is "bad," but stepping into that area could be what you need. During sex, it could mean letting your partner take you with more abandon and strength.

5. Surrender to what happens

A lot of the disconnection during sex can come from the pressure of achieving something. This could mean having an orgasm, trying to look good, or being seen as good in bed. It will distract you from the beauty and sacredness of the moment. Maybe you should look at the outcome as experiencing this moment with your partner. If you weren't pressured into reaching a milestone while being intimate, how deeper could your relationship go, and surrender to your partner?

Chapter 5: Taking Care of Your Body

Taking care of yourself is number one when it comes to releasing your sexuality. If you don't make sure you are taken care of then how will you be able to understand what you really want? So, in this chapter, we will look at a 20-step plan that is full of tips on revamping yourself without don't anything extreme. These are all things that you can implement every day.

1. *Begin your day with a cup of warm lemon water*

Get rid of coffee first thing in the morning and instead, choose a cup of warm water with a teaspoon of apple cider vinegar, and the juice of half a lemon. This will help to improve your digestion; kick starts your metabolism and will make your liver very happy. It also gives you a hydration boosts, and alkalizes your system, unlike caffeine, which tends to dehydrate you and is acidic. Caffeine also tends to exhausts your liver and ups your levels of cortisol, which may end up leading your body's inability to get rid of toxins, or burn fat.

2. *Have water to drink all day*

The water that you drink needs to be room temperature or warm, or at least warm enough so that body doesn't have use energy to warm it up before it becomes hydrating and beneficial. It also helps to purge out toxins and up your elimination. Hydration is the most important thing when it comes to health and vitality; after all, the body is made up of 75% water. If you find yourself bored with regular water, try infusing it. Some of the best combinations are cucumber and basil, peach and sage, and strawberry and mint.

3. *Start your day with greens and some meditation*

Instead of bacon and eggs, go for a green smoothie or green juice for breakfast to give you the vitamin boost you need. Also, you can try meditation. Simply try to focus on your breathing for at least one to five minutes. It's best if you can do this for 15 to 20. You can either do both or one of them.

4. *Relax*

Take some time out of your day to relax. Get comfy and watch a movie or read a book you've been meaning to.

5. *Say no to sugar*

Skip over sugar and choose to drink healing herbal tea during your day. Teas will provide you with antioxidants and are a lot more satisfying. Peppermint and vanilla are great options. If you don't want warm tea, make a big batch of tea and refrigerate it for refreshing iced tea.

6. *Use affirmations*

Write down your favorite affirmations on some sticky notes and stick them to different places around your house like the bathroom mirror or fridge; places that you see frequently. Repeat these affirmations to yourself throughout the day.

7. *Use walnuts as your snack of choice*

They will not only curb your hunger, but they will give you brain power! Walnuts are one of the few foods out there that are prehistoric, and they contain good amounts of omega-3 fatty acids, which you can normally only find in fish. They also stimulate your nervous system and brain.

8. *Read things that inspire you*

Find some articles on websites and blogs that are inspiring to your read them during the day.

9. Chew

Chewing your food well is crucial for good digestion, and that also goes for healthy waistline and weight. A goal is to chew each bite 30 times. Since your day is so relaxing, you can definitely make more of an effort to chew more.

10. Eat in a peaceful location

When you eat, make sure you are in a peaceful place. You should try to do this every time you eat, but just choosing certain days to do this can help as well. The peacefulness will help you to eat more mindfully and make you more conscious of how you eat.

11. Dream big

Write out your three biggest and three smallest goals as everything sits right now.

12. Are you feeling creative?

Create yourself a vision board. Find images on the internet or in magazines to create a collage of images that will remind you of your dreams and goals in life. Make sure you place it where you can view it every day. Visualize these things actually happening. This has been proven to be a very powerful manifesting tool.

13. Burn some incense

Pick your favorite incense and burn it in your house to help boost your mood. White sage is a great choice.

14. Drink a fresh juice of lemon, ginger, celery, beetroot, and carrot

This drink will provide you with a boost of energy and is delicious. This drink contains the lots of minerals and vitamins.

15. Take a bubble bath and spoil yourself a bit

Use every little thing in your bath. Use candles, bath salts, bath bubbles, and aromatherapy. Make sure if you want to use candles that they are non-toxic. Pick candles with vegetable wax, beeswax, or soy wax.

16. Try some low-key exercises

Connect yourself with nature by taking a walk. Walk barefoot on the grass or on the beach. This is a perfect way to get some vitamin D. You can also do some stretching or yoga. This will boost your endorphins and boost your immune system and spirit.

17. Take a nap

Take yourself a nap and don't even feel guilty about it.

18. Cook

Try something new. Make a healthy recipe that you have been interested in trying for a while.

19. Laugh

Turn the TV to a funny show or call up your best friend. Laughing is the best medicine and is amazing for your soul. It will help you to feel better and put you in a good mood.

20. Use lavender

Make use of lavender oil. Place a bit on your temples to help yourself relax and calm down after a long day.

Chapter 6: Improving Romance

Studies have found that men are still initiating sex twice as much as women. Considering the liberated times we live in, why? Research has found that the more often either people in a relationship initiates, the happier the both are towards each other. Everybody loves to be seduced, and you initiating will send a huge signal to your significant other: I find you attractive. I want you. I desire you.

If you don't suggest sex, then how will your partner know that you're not just having sex with them to make them happy? The answer is that they don't know that, and many women are aware this problem.

So why is that women are still the ones say yes instead of asking for it? The most common answer is that "men typically get to it first." But there are many other reasons out there.

Women tend to become more bored with monogamy than men do. In a German study, they found that at the beginning of a relationship, on average, the men and women had about equal desire for each other. Jump forward a while, and things begin to change. The women take a sharp dive after they have been with their partners for one to four years, but the same doesn't happen to the men.

Men have a head start when it comes to sex drive because of their testosterone, which is the hormone that boosts sex drive. When it comes to women, they have a lose-lose scenario. They don't initiate because the sex drive will drop while in a long-term relationship, and their libidos don't receive a boost because they don't take charge. When you initiate sex, you receive a libido boost, and men are the ones that get this boost, and they are ones that need it the least.

Society makes everybody think that it's the man's job. Another huge belief is that women on turned on by their partner wanting them. They need a man to "throw them around the bedroom" and "take charge;" in other words, be the initiators.

Nobody would argue that it isn't a turn on. Everybody wants to have sex with a person that desires us. But if a woman doesn't ever initiate, then they don't get the erotic power surge from initiating. It's sexier to be the one that asks for sex, than the one that submits.

Submission has its place in being erotic as well if you are playing out a fantasy scene from *Fifty Shades*. It isn't as sexy when the submission comes with a stifled yawn and resigned nod when his hand rubs down your thigh as you about to go to sleep.

Women don't initiate because they are afraid of rejection. Women seem to love blaming their self. If their partner quits initiating sex, they believe they have done something wrong. They're not good in bed; they're not sexy, they're too fat. They constantly worry about taking charge and initiating sex to their partner in case their partner doesn't want sex. They believe their partner just doesn't want sex with them.

There have you have some of the reasons why women choose not to initiate sex and the positives that can happen when they do. If you tend to be more passive, and you are looking to change your sex life, then there is one thing you can do.

How to Initiate Sex

There is no need to act like a porn star to inform your partner that you're in the mood, but you should…

Make sure that you have clear signals. These are some things that could happen if your signals aren't clear: he may not understand that you're suggesting sex and completely misses the signal. You end up angry and feeling rejected; he didn't even understand that you were up for sex.

When you're not clear, it can leave both of you in a very bad place of trying to figure out which expressions and touches are just affection and which are signals for sex. In an ideal situation, you would both talk to each other and figure out a specific signal.

There is no need to be blatant. It can start with a kiss that lasts longer than normal with some tongue action. You stroke partner in an area near his sexual zone to see the kind of response that you get, or you could slip him a sexy note in his pocket before he goes off to work detailing things that you would like to do that night.

You could invite him to your shower or bath, or you could tell him that when you wear a certain article of clothing that it means you are up for sex. There are some couples that use fridge magnets that they move to indicate how interested they are in sex for the day.

Tread lightly when initiating if he has stopped wanting sex. Is there a chance that he doesn't just want less sex, but no sex? There is a big divide in opinion as to whether a woman should try to tempt a man into sex by doing suggestive things such as opening the door wearing nothing by heels.

The main reason there is a divide is that this can work for some mean, and it can freak others out. The kind of reaction you get from him will depend on the reasons why he isn't interested in sex.

If he as slipped into seeing you as a friend instead of a lover, then shocking him into viewing you as a sex object could be what he needs. If he is staying away from sex because of erection problems, then the pressure of you wanting him and him not being able to perform could be a disaster. This can cause his sexual confidence to fall.

Another way that this could backfire is that sex is too available to them. So, when you push sex at him, he will turn you down. This is the same reason why some weight loss experts will tell you to fill up your house with cakes and chocolates: the more available they are to you, the less you are going to want it.

Talk to each other honestly about why he is having libido problems instead of jumping into something you once saw in a B-grade movie.

It's Not About You

So maybe you have stuck your neck out there, and he knocked you back? This doesn't mean you did it wrong, or what you did was unsexy. There are a lot of reasons why a man may not want sex.

Work with him to look at his lifestyle. Maybe he needs to get more sleep, reduce stress, exercise, stop smoking, or cut back on alcohol. Maybe he needs to go to the doctor because of low testosterone levels or is having erection problems. It's far more likely that he has a problem as to why he is saying no than it is about you.

Chapter 7: Sexual Anatomy

If a woman's private parts had a Facebook page, her relationship status would be "it's complicated." After all, research has found only 26% of women have ever looked closely are their private parts. Guys have it a lot easier. Their stuff is there waiting to be experienced. Most of a woman's parts are internal, so it's a bit harder so what they've got.

Here's a bit of an incentive, the more you pay attention to your vagina, the more pleasure you will have. Women that are more positive about their genitals tend to be more comfortable with their self, more likely to experiment in bed, and have better chances of orgasms.

Investigation

First off, the vagina is not the complete genital area. If you look at yourself naked in a full-length mirror, you will see your vulva, which is the outside portion of your privates. Think of them as a movie cast: The supporting actor is your vulva, and the marquee stars are the G-spot and clitoris. Every part is there for entertainment and for your sexual needs, but to get the best performance, you have to make sure all of them get some love. So, close and lock your door, take off your shoes, and grab yourself a mirror.

Before spreading your legs, you are able to see the pubic mound and the labia majora. These parts contain fatty tissue that protects the vagina and clitoris. Pleasure reception is normally weak in this area, but some play can up the signal.

When you push apart the outer lips, you will find the labia minora. This area is full of secreting glands, nerve endings, and blood vessels. They aren't the only thing providing lube. When you spread them apart, you will find the Bartholin's glands. These are actually microscopic, so you won't actually be able to see them. There is a gland on either side of the vaginal opening. The glands begin to lubricate the vaginal canal when you become aroused. They normally on release a little bit of moisture, which is one of the reasons why a woman needs a lot of foreplay in order for them to stay wet.

The little pink nub that is about the size of a pencil eraser is your clitoris, and her only job is sexual pleasure. There are about 8,000 nerve endings in the clitoris, the largest number that can be found in the whole body and double the number of nerves in the penis. You knew she was sensitive, but you may not know that she has legs. All you see is the head, but there is a body that looks like a wishbone, called crura, which goes three inches into the vagina, located just under the pubic mound and leads to the G-spot.

The best way to stimulate the clitoris is consistent, direct, and gentle manual or oral stimulation. Friction often feels amazing, but this little start can be a little overexposed. When you reach climax, the clitoris will swell, which can cause friction to become painful. Most of the time you can lighten up on the stimulation, and it will feel good again.

When your clitoris becomes overly sensitive, it is telling you to let the vagina have some fun. This is the four to seven inches canal; size varies among women, can't hold a candle to your clitoris when it comes to nerve endings. It does boast some nerve endings. Within the first couple of inches, there are hundreds of nerve endings and are sensitive. Try shorter, shallow thrusts to stimulate these nerves.

Moving deeper into your vaginal walls, you will find the G-spot. Not all women are able to use its potential, but if you can the reward is amazing. It's a spongy area the size of a nickel and is found about an inch into the anterior wall of the vagina. It will feel knotty and bumpy striations that are similar to a walnut and likes a hands-on, tough-love approach. You have to be turned on before you can find it because the tissue doesn't swell until after proper foreplay.

If you've never had a G-spot orgasm, don't worry. Just so you know, G-spot orgasms are often deep and expansive, while clitoris orgasms feel intense and acute. Most of the time women aren't going to say they had a G-spot orgasm, but instead, it works more as an enhancer to their orgasm. Everything works together. So, as long as you have an orgasm, that's all that matters.

Myths

Let's debunk some myths about the female genitals.

1. *It smells bad*

This is the most irritating myth because it can keep women from enjoying and accepting oral sex. Women tend to be insecure about the smell of the vagina, and this is mainly due to douche advertisements that make people believe vaginas are supposed to smell like rosewater. FYI, they don't. Everybody has their own scent, but most have a musky scent that men are wired to be attracted to.

2. *All of them look alike*

Like all parts of the body, the vulva and vagina have basic shapes, but there are variations with pubic hair, symmetry, and coloration. The labia minora tends to have the biggest difference between women.

3. It's too loose or too tight

Unless a woman is still a virgin, or they have gone through a traumatic birthing experience with multiple births, there isn't going to be a huge anatomical difference in the vaginal canal. The feeling of looseness or tightness has to do with lubrication. If you're really wet, then there won't be much friction. If you're too dry, then there will be too much friction. It's helpful to have a tube of lube on hand.

4. Things can get lost

For some reason, women tend to think that it's a never-ending tube. It's more like a sock. It only goes so far, so you are able to pull anything out. The cervix is microscopic, and sperm is the only thing that can slip through.

Chapter 8: Working Past Sexual Difficulty

Sexual dysfunction is a problem during any phase of a person's sexual cycle that will prevent the person from being satisfied from any sexual activity. A person's sexual response cycle includes four phases:

- The first is excitement
- The second is plateau
- The third is orgasm
- The fourth is resolution

Some causes of sexual dysfunction might include:

Physical causes

Many medical or physical conditions could cause problems with a person's sexual function. Some conditions are drug abuse, alcoholism, liver or kidney failure, menopause, hormonal imbalances, neurological disorders, heart disease, and diabetes. The side effects of medicines like antidepressants could affect sexual function and desire.

Psychological causes

These can include anxiety, stress from work, relationship or marital problems, past sexual trauma, feelings of guilt, depression, and concern about sexual performance.

The most common problems women have with sexual dysfunction are:

Inhibited sexual desire

This includes lack of interest in sex or sexual desire. There are many factors that could contribute to lack of desire like fatigue, stress, pregnancy, depression, chemotherapy, cancer, and hormonal changes. Boredom with regular sex routines can also contribute to not having the desire for sex just like lifestyle factors like caring for children and career.

Inability to get aroused

Not being able to be aroused during sex could include insufficient vaginal lubrication. Not being able to be aroused can be related to inadequate stimulation or anxiety. Researchers are studying how blood flow problems can affect the clitoris and vagina. This can cause arousal problems.

Anorgasmia or Lack of orgasm

This is the absence or delay of orgasm. It could be caused by lack of knowledge, inexperience, sexual inhibition and psychological factors like abuse, sexual trauma, anxiety, and guilt. Other factors include chronic diseases, medicines, and insufficient stimulation.

Intercourse that's painful

This can be caused by many problems like sexually transmitted diseases, scar tissue from surgery, poor lubrication, inflammation of the vagina, ovarian cysts, pelvic mass, and endometriosis. One condition vaginismus is involuntary, painful muscle spasms that are around the entrance to the vagina. This occurs in women who have a fear that penetration is going to be painful. It might also come from a phobia about sex or from previous traumatic experiences.

Sexual dysfunction is diagnosed by first doing a physical exam along with evaluating the symptoms. The doctor will do a pelvic exam the see how healthy the reproductive organs are along with a Pap test to see if there are any changes in the cervix. They could order other tests to rule out all problems that could be a contributing factor to this dysfunction.

They will evaluate the person's attitudes toward sex along with other factors like drug abuse, alcohol, relationship problems, past trauma or sexual abuse, anxiety, and fear. This will help the doctor find the cause of the problem and take appropriate actions to treat it.

Sexual dysfunction is treated with a team effort between trained therapists, health care providers, and patient. Many types of sexual dysfunction get corrected by treating the psychological or physical problems. Other treatments could focus on:

- *Giving education* – Educating the patient about the human anatomy, sexual function, and changes that are normal with aging and other sexual responses and behaviors might help women overcome their anxiety about sexual performance and functions.

- *Enhancing stimulation* – This could include using erotic materials like books and videos, changes in sexual routines, and masturbation.

- *Providing distraction techniques* – Non-erotic or erotic fantasies, music, exercises involving intercourse, television or videos might be used to help with relaxation and get rid of anxiety.

- *Encouraging non-coital behavior* – Non-coital behaviors like any physically stimulating activity that doesn't involve sex like massage is used to give comfort and increase communication with partners.

- *Minimizing pain* – Learning sexual positions that let the woman control how deep the penetration is can help relieve pain. Using lubricants can reduce pain due to friction. Taking a warm bath before having sex could also help with relaxation.

Chapter 9: Improving Your Relationship

Think about being in a relationship with somebody that you didn't love. You felt like this person was not good enough for you, worthless, and flawed. You thought you could never leave this relationship. You are stuck. What type of relationship would this be? How will it affect your life, behavior, and thoughts?

For people that were raised in a home that shamed their children, that was constantly told you aren't good enough. The relationship we have with ourselves is based on the messages we received as a child. If you believe that you aren't good enough, you will feel uncomfortable in your skin. You will only feel comfortable if you spend time with people that encourage our discomfort.

Most anybody could give you examples of things that happened to them during their childhood. A friend once told me a story of when she was in the 5th grade and was in the school spelling bee. She was the top three in her class and moved on to the countywide competition for that grade level. She was the best speller that I knew. There were words I couldn't pronounce that she could spell. What always amazed me was words that I knew she knew how to spell she would spell wrong. It was like she would spell the word wrong just so she wouldn't get first place. In everything, she did it was that way. I finally asked her when we were in eighth grade why she did it. She answered with she didn't know what I was talking about. I told her what I had witnessed her doing like spelling a word wrong or slowing down, so she didn't cross the finish line first. She looked at me confused and denied ever doing those things. I knew she grew up in a home where her parents didn't encourage her as mine did. I was never great at anything, but my parents encouraged me in everything I did. She was great with everything she did but didn't get the encouragement she needed and deserved. I honestly think she thought she wasn't good enough to be first and would subconsciously sabotage herself so she would never be first.

If you would like a good reference point for dealing with low self-esteem check out the poem *Success Through a Positive Mental Attitude* by Napoleon Hill. It is my go to when I start to feel down on myself.

If you carry around a message that you don't think you are enough, you are going to create so many obstacles that will be greater than anything life will ever throw at you. I sometimes think of my friend and wonder how much simpler her life would have been if she hadn't carried around that burden. I look around me at all the success and wish I could give some to my friend. She has struggled her whole life. She is always critical of others because she can see their flaws but they are successful, and she isn't.

She was raised in a home where it was never okay to not be perfect and make mistakes. She was never allowed to be a kid. She had to learn as she went. She was szxchamed and criticized for everything she tried to do. Her mother constantly told her she was never good enough.

I remember an incident when we were around the age of 15. I was spending the night with her, and we were riding with her father to go pick up her mom from work. We were sitting in the back seat of the car, and her father was pumping gas. A man in his 20s walked by and waved. We both smiled and waved back. Her mom whirled around and looked at my friend with a scowl on her face and asked her sarcastically, "Do you honestly think he was waving at you?" She bowed her head and shook her head no. I just looked at her mom dumbfounded. My mother never talked to me that way. I don't know if her mom was thinking the man was waving to her and not my friend and I or if she was just so used to putting my friend down, it was now second nature to her mom to just automatically put her down. I honestly think it was the latter. Her missile has struck my friend, and her message sank home. My friend honestly thought from that day forward that there wasn't a man alive who would think she was attractive.

When you have been raised this way, and you get into an adult relationship, you are lost, to begin with. You enter this relationship weak, longing for love that you have never gotten, and desperate. You are primed for being targeted by your emotional manipulator since your radar is off and you can't see reality as reality is.

To quote Robert Burney from Dance of the Wounded Soul, "Toxic shame is the belief that there is something inherently wrong with who we are, with our being. Guilt is, I made a mistake. I did something wrong. Toxic shame is, I am a mistake. There is something wrong with me."

Everyone is born good enough. We don't need anybody's acceptance or permission to be good enough. Those toxic message we get from others are messages that the got from other toxic people, and the cycle goes back for generations. It is a disease that will get passed down until somebody wakes up and heals themselves before they pass it down further.

When you are an adult, no one can give you the realization that you are good enough. This is something that we must wake up within ourselves. It begins by being aware there is a problem. Once we are aware of it, we can watch it in our behaviors, thoughts, and actions. We can look at it as a spectator.

Once we realize the relationship we are having with ourselves is toxic, we can then realize that our relationships with others we sabotaged by these patterns and frequencies that we are accustomed to. We won't be able to have healthy relationships until we get healthy.

When we have gained awareness, we must begin to change our internal message. Be kind to yourself is something codependents find extremely difficult to do. We are used to being blamed for everything, and we think we aren't good enough. These messages have been ingrained in us, but we must begin changing this message. Once we realize what we are doing, we must be mindful of how we process information that we receive. If your significant other begins to yell at you, think about what you might have done to warrant this attack. You are allowed to make mistakes without being yelled at.

Be mindful of what you allow in and how you interpret what comes at you.

Look at people around you who are successful and realize they aren't perfect. Then realize you don't have to be perfect either. If you want to try something, do something, or be something, you don't have to be perfect. Give yourself permission to do what you have always been shamed for. You will surprise yourself at just how liberated you will feel.

The way you process information has to change. Feeling like everybody is better than you have to change. We must train ourselves to look at clues differently. Instead of looking for why everything is our fault, we need to begin seeing situations with a discerning eye and focusing on the truth.

Turning our eyes outward while being mindful of how we see our environment and be aware that you were taught to make bad judgments about ourselves. It might look like a huge task, but you will begin to see reality from the fiction you have been led to believe.

Find a reason to live a healthier lifestyle than you should. Find a reason to eat better or exercise that doesn't center on obligation. Think about how lucky you are to be able to do these things. If you like to run, be grateful. If you like lifting weights, reflect on every improvement. Give attention to every milestone you reach. Soon you won't be thinking that you should but what you can get to.

Imperfections were never meant to be controlled. Trying to be perfect can encompass your existence. You need to realize that your imperfections were never meant to be controlled. You absolutely cannot fight genetics. You must learn to embrace what you have been given. You might fight it, but you must learn to love the body you were given at birth and the sooner you can do that the better.

I have never been happy with my body, and it pisses me off most days. When thinking about it as a relationship, I must treat it like I want to be treated in a relationship. Instead of trying to manipulate ourselves into what we aren't, we need to let go of the control and practice acceptance. If we can do this, it will lead to things like being happy that our clothes fit a bit too tight. If we can't do it, it will lead to obsessively exercising and restrictive eating.

We need to practice self-care. Let's go back to relationships. How do you want to be treated? Treat yourself with the love, dignity, and respect you deserve. Listen to what your body wants and needs. Bad self-care can indicate that something deeper is happening either with your priorities or emotionally. Talk to yourself like you would in any given relationship to understand what is going on.

Love the gray areas. I'm not a fan of black vs. white or good vs. bad. I work on two ends of the spectrum, and either can be damaging.

Find a middle ground. Embrace balance. If you only have the time to exercise three days, that's fine. If you can only exercise for 30 minutes each day, that's fine, too. Find your balance. Stop trying to live on each end of the spectrum. Exercising every day for hours and not exercising at all is both bad for you.

Never put yourself down. Think about a good relationship. Do you insult and put your partner down? Do they do that to you? Do you tell them their flaws? Do they point out yours? I'm hoping all of you are answering now. Think of your body as your friend. You need to love your friend. Understand that through everything, you are enough.

Chapter 10: Going Beyond the Bedroom

You have been working what seems like forever. You are tired by the time you get home. You are excited to see your partner, and you have some fun planned for the night. When you sit down on the couch, you get an overwhelming feeling of exhaustion. You fall asleep. There are ways to include sex in your daily routine. The couch might seduce you into going to sleep; you could find the energy and time to seduce your partner or vice versa successfully. Most experts say sex is essential to keeping a romantic, healthy relationship.

Keeping sex and love alive is what keeps the relationship alive. It is just like the roots of a tree. To keep the energy flowing and the sap rising, you must provide things that are interesting and new. Seduction is as simple as making your partner ask what you have done to make yourself so energized. When you are seductive and enthusiastic, you are the most attractive of your lover.

How can you stop the couch from seducing you into slumber especially when the temps are getting colder, and that blanket is calling your name? Here are some ways to bring sex back into your daily routine:

Spontaneity is Key

Being spontaneous is the key. Have a quickie at lunch, don't skip on foreplay. Foreplay begins with simple things like caressing, kissing, and touching everything you can reach. Have sex before you ever get out of bed, during breaks, during lunch, or after work. If you don't' work together and can't meet that often, surprise your partner at their job to add some excitement. FaceTime them during the day to build up suspense.

Predictability is the number one killer of passion. With time, we know every single move our partner will make. They have also memorized ours. The key is breaking the predictability factor. Couples fall into routines. They will only have sex at night or on the weekend. Shake things up. Take a break from putting the dishes up. It won't feel so much like a chore after you have made love. If you feel the "urge" in the middle of a movie, press stop and finish it later. Delight and surprise your mate with unpredictability.

Take Time for a Morning Quickie

Grab your morning beverage of choice and jump back into bed for a quickie with a partner or favorite toy. Morning sex is a great way to begin your day on the right foot.

Shower Together Because You Both Need One

You must put the energy and time and make an effort to keep the passion in a relationship. When intimacy and touch are put on a back burner, other things get put there, too. Make an effort to continue to connect and physically touch. You could wake up earlier a few times each week and have sex or join your partner in the shower.

Midday Phone Sex

There are ways to add sex to your daily routine with or without your partner. Phone sex can happen anytime, anywhere. It is creative and unexpected and a great way to enjoy sex anytime during the day. Your partner will be surprised by this call.

Try Sexting

Don't have to time or freedom to talk? Send a quick sext. Closeness and intimacy don't have to be a physical act. It is an emotionally intimate act. Sending dirty pics and sexting might keep the fires burning.

Have Sex Somewhere Other Than the Bedroom

Spontaneous sex out of the bedroom will break the pattern of predictability and changes the monotony of daily chores into an exciting adventure. Try a department store changing room or restaurant bathroom. There are many options available to give your sex life a boost. You only need imagination. The goal is to find opportunities to duplicate the heat of a budding relationship and put the passion back into your established relationship.

Kiss Like You Mean It

You can incorporate sex into your daily routine. This doesn't mean you have to do the deed every single day. Make an effort just to kiss and touch passionately. We aren't talking pecks on the cheeks here. You need to do this daily to make you feel connected to your partner. Having sex regularly can have the same effect. Make it a regular part of your weekly routine.

Have a Date with a Vibrator

Taking a lunch break with a vibrator or sex toy is a wonderful way to change up your workday. It also helps to relieve stress fast.

Do Some Research to Get New Ideas

There is something to be said about being a life partner. Apply this to your sex life. Read about sexual techniques and try out what you find with your partner. Change up the way you touch, where you touch and your physical moves. Explore different ways to get fluent in the language of love.

Give a Massage at Bedtime

Head to bed with a wonderful, sexual massage. Get touched and be touched.

Do Things You Wanted to do at the Beginning of Your Relationship

Romance gets blown out of proportion in this culture. It is fleeting and momentary. It adds excitement to the relationship, but it isn't your way of life. You can't continue to keep it happening with all the stress of your daily life. It is a useful tool to let each other know you still love each other. If there is a lack of excitement or romance, recharge this connection and have a celebration about your mutual desire, affection, and love with these rituals:

1. Pick one evening every week to have a date night. Do things you did when you began dating.

2. Have a romantic picnic in a secluded spot or breakfast in bed.

3. Send your partner a card, cologne, flowers, a plant, or something they would enjoy just because to show them they are special.

4. Take a class in something you both enjoy like cooking, swimming, sailing, stained glass, painting, pottery, rollerblading, acting, skiing, or dancing. Get involved in the community to make new memories.

5. When your partner feels down, arrange a surprise, present, date, tell them a joke or give them a hug.

6. Meet at a bar and pick each other up.

7. Take a vacation to your favorite romantic spot.

Sex needs to be your number one priority for both you and your partner or you if you are single. It will keep the candle burning bright and has health benefits which shouldn't be ignored.

If you find your sexual energy has left you, there are ways you can harness it to get it flowing again. Add these tips to your daily to-do list to help improve your relationships, quality of life, health, and overall enjoyment of living. Life is meant to be fun, and human sexuality is the most fun part of it.

Here are some things you can do to help you reconnect with your sexual energy:

1. *Get naked*: Yes, it is that simple. Being constantly covered by clothing can make you forget about your sexuality. There is no better reminder than getting naked. When you are naked, you will move differently. You will be more graceful and softer with yourself. This can put you in touch with your femininity, and this will put you in touch with your sexuality.

2. *Love your body*: This is two-fold. First, find specific things about your body that you love. Everyone's body is different. No two bodies are alike. Everyone is unique physically, and this should make you feel wonderful. Take time to admire these things about your body and let the sexual energy flow. Second, loving your body means you need to take care of it. This means you should eat right and try to exercise.

You can honor your body by doing this. There isn't anything sexier than a healthy body.

3. *Flirt:* This is something I love to do, but I don't do it often enough. Flirting is energizing and fun for everyone involved. This can charge your sexual energy, and you can use it anytime you need to. Send your partner a romantic text while they are at work. It will have a positive effect on them and you, too. It can instantly change your mood into a happy one.

4. *Laugh:* Laughter is a powerful tool in many ways. It aids in making sexual energy. Laughter can get you out of your head and into your body since you can feel the physical effects of the laughter. It makes you feel marvelous. I love to laugh. I would love to be able to laugh all day long.

5. *Dress:* Your clothing of choice will have a large effect on if you can get and keep your sexual energy flowing. You don't have to wear what others think is sexy. As long as you think you look sexy, is all that matters. Make sure you feel comfortable in your clothes.

That's it. Take all of these things into consideration to get back to feeling sexual and see the benefits of what tapping into your sexual energy can do for you and your partner. Use it daily to get the most benefits.

Chapter 11: Foreplay

Foreplay is a basic necessity for a woman. Let's compare a woman with a car. Do you just start your car and take off every morning? Absolutely not. You have to let it warm up. If you don't, you might cause problems for your motor.

This all holds true for women, too. You must warm her up. When you have her all warmed and lubed up, she will rev up and go for hours. She will only stop when you turn your engine off.

Instead of whining about foreplay like it is some excruciating ordeal or a waiting game before you actually get what you want. Look at it as if it was the key to an extremely gratifying sexual experience.

Women are very emotional creatures and are looking for intimacy and appreciation from their partners. They aren't mechanical objects to just switch off and on when you want them.

You must know women and what they need to get the most from your relationship. It works both ways.

If you can give them what they need, you will get yours plus a bonus without even asking for it.

There isn't a manual to tell you how to give women foreplay. There isn't a step by step guide on how to give foreplay that she actually needs. It's easy if you can change your goal from just sticking it in and getting off.

Everyone has five senses. You need to learn how to use all of them.

You have the sense of hearing, taste, sight, smell, and touch. You need to learn to appreciate and get creative. Just a simple wink can put a light in her eyes since it shows her you think she is beautiful.

Do not rush foreplay. Rub her, smell her, suck her, touch her, lick her, kiss her, pay attention to each part of her body to get her wound up.

Don't give her less than she deserves. Never rush her. You must wait until she is begging you to take her. This is the sign you need to look for to know that you have satisfied her completely. When you can satisfy your woman, she will begin to treat you like a god.

Foreplay is an essential need for women. She needs a warm up to get ready for sex, not just physically but emotionally and mentally, too.

Give your woman plenty of foreplay, and you will see your sex life improve drastically. The more foreplay, the more chances of giving her multiple orgasms. The more orgasms she has, the more she is going to want sex. This is why foreplay is so important.

Take time to master foreplay and how to please her in every sexual way. Learn to be an expert lover. The type of man who truly knows what a woman needs and wants. A man who understands her sexuality and can please her in every emotional and sexual way. Be the man every woman wants.

Here are some tips on foreplay:

Treat her like an appetizer and always get one. Couples forget about foreplay completely and just go straight for sex. By doing this, they are setting themselves up for failure. By performing the right foreplay can take sex from a zero to 1,000 on the horny scale.

Sexual satisfaction and foreplay go hand in hand for women. Women need foreplay for sex to be good. That is a great reason not to cut corners. Foreplay is so important for women because it takes them longer to get in the mood. Women complain that men will skip the foreplay and go straight for sex. Women need that time to open up. Foreplay will help their natural lubrication flow and makes sex more pleasurable.

Sensuality is the key to good foreplay. Holding hands, caressing each other's arms, legs, hair, nearness by having your head on his shoulders. This will help to build sexual arousal and tension.

Continue foreplay during sex. Don't just do it before. Don't rush from touching straight to sex. Foreplay needs to be lingered over. It is usually the longest part of the whole sexual encounter. Foreplay has a bad name since it sounds like something that gets started and then just stops. All the seduction, touching and talking need to continue through the whole sex process.

To try to save time, couples try to be more efficient with sex by stopping foreplay altogether. Many get lazy about foreplay as their relationship progresses. This is when efficiency sets in. The mindset goes to just get the orgasm over with. It gets so shortened that takes the pleasure completely out of it.

Don't ignore the rest of the body with foreplay. People just head straight for the erogenous zones when they hop into bed. That all and well, but there are other body parts that like to be touched, too. Touching these will help to build up the excitement. The mistake most people make is they jump right to the genitals and ignore her earlobes, neck, face and everywhere else.

Savor the entire body instead of just trying to get her aroused by kissing and heading straight for sex. Learn where your woman's erogenous zones are. Then wait before you do anything with them. Don't go for them right away. Let the anticipation build. Learn to tease her.

Talk about what you want. Communication is the key to foreplay both before and during sex. Talk about what you want. Don't just sit there and be polite. Have a sexual conversation with her about what you like. Do this when you aren't under stress or worried about criticism. Continue to talk about it. One conversation isn't going to cover it. Check in with each other over time. Just because something worked last night, doesn't mean it will work tonight. Give your partner feedback during the moment. During foreplay let them know what feels good and what doesn't.

Foreplay isn't what you would expect. Learn to think outside the box when it comes to foreplay. Most of us focus on "fooling around, " but there are other things that serve as foreplay. It could be as simple as holding hands. You could also do a striptease, dress up in a sexy outfit, do some dirty dancing, or massage. Flirting can also be foreplay. Giving a shoulder massage just might be what your woman needs to relax her. Other forms of foreplay like oral sex is always a great turn on. Don't forget all those little tidbits that get you in the mood as well.

Foreplay is just as important as sex. Some think it is more important than sex especially women. Many women need a lot of foreplay since they are multitaskers and do many things at one time. Getting in the mood for sex is not easy for them.

If they are thinking about finances, children, household chores, and what needs to be done, foreplay allows them to get out of their own heads and into the mindset of sex.

Foreplay isn't just for women even though they need it more; men enjoy it as much as women do. If you can add these moves to your routine, you will win the trophy for best foreplay ever.

1. While giving your man oral sex, wrap your hands around his shaft and use the other to massage and tug on his "boys."

2. Just like they need to learn your sweet spots, discover their sweet spots as well. When you know what makes them moan, suck or nibble on it while making out or while playing with them. You will be sending electricity straight to their manhood. They will soon be standing at attention.

3. Begin foreplay before you get to the bedroom. While eating dinner take his hand and slide it under your skirt or take yours and play with his member to keep his mind of what is about to happen.

4. Get adventurous and tie him up. Then get dominant and order him to do something erotic to you like giving you oral sex.

5. Many women don't pay attention to men's nipples. Take the time and treat them just like you want yours treated. They are just like yours after all.

6. Pleasure yourself while he watches. Order him not to touch you unless you ask him to. It will show him how you liked to be touched so he can give you everything you want.

7. While making out, suck on his fingers to show him what is in store for him later.

8. While giving him oral sex, arch your back and stick your butt in the air. It will make you look like a pin-up girl and gives him an incredible view of your body.

9. If you need to use lube, rub it on his manhood slowly and erotically. Have him put some in his hand and place it on you. It will make sex feel hotter than ever.

Chapter 12: Passion Boosting Sex Positions

At some point in your sex life, you are going to realize you need less raunch and more romance. With lives being busy, it is easy getting caught up in the same old routines and that means that we don't put every effort into making the best times with our partners.

Just taking it slow and looking into each other's eyes can make a world of difference. Having that type of connection with your partner has been proven to improve orgasms.

The best sex is like having a conversation with your bodies. It is important to connect to your partner during sex by having as much eye contact as you possibly can. Having connection during sex will transcend into deeper levels or orgasms. By having a spiritual connection as well as animal instincts during sex, make a world of difference.

Here are the best positions to help maintain a longer, passionate sexual session. All of these sex positions, if done right, could bring couples closer.

The Rocking Horse

The best way to add romance to your relationship is making eye contact. Keeping this in mind, any position where you can look at your partner will make it more passionate.

The man will sit cross-legged and leans back. He will support himself with his arms behind him or lean against a wall. You will kneel over him hugging him with your thighs. Lower yourself at your own pace and penetrate yourself at the depth you like. This position allows you to adjust your body so you can stimulate your clitoris. This position is great as it allows you to look into each other's eyes and you can kiss each other's nipples and necks.

The Nirvana

This is a variation of the missionary position. This is a favorite because it is sexy, intimate, and easy.

You just lie on your back and your partner climbs on top of you. He will place his legs on either side of yours. He will penetrate you slowly. If penetration is too hard this way, he can penetrate you normally then bring his legs out from between yours. In this position, he can thrust away as you meet each of his thrusts with your pelvis.

Ask your partner to kiss and touch you. You can also play with his rear and run your fingers up and down his back for wonderful sensations.

The Padlock

This next position is more adventurous. You will need to have a kitchen counter, sink, or chair handy. The man will hold his woman like she has just jumped into his arms. You can be sitting on the edge of the bed or kitchen counter.

You will wrap your legs around his waist and wrap your arms around his neck. This position allows slow movements, romantic swaying, and passionate kisses. He can grab your butt and lift you as you thrust your hips against him. This allows you to be naughty and sensual. You can whisper your naughty thought into his ears. Tell him exactly what you are feeling.

For a variation, you could lean back to gain extra depth.

The Suspender

If your man gets tired during Ascent, he can rest himself against a wall. You will get more energy by bending your legs so they are against the wall. You can use this as leverage to bounce yourself up and down. Your man can use his hands to lift you as well. Working together to make this a romantic and rhythmical session.

For a variation, have him turn you around so your back is against the wall. This way he can penetrate you deeper.

Close Up

Spooning is wonderful, but it gets better when you have sex during it. Even without eye contact, your man can kiss your neck and whisper all the dirty things he is going to do to you. This gives him a feeling of dominance, while you stay submissive.

You both lay on your sides with your man behind you. He will enter you from behind. You need to push your backside toward him as you arch your back. He has the opportunity to reach around and play with your breasts. You can reach back and put your hands on his hips or butt and enjoy feeling him thrusting in and out of you.

Zen Pause

Mix up the close up by flipping on your side so you are facing each other. Hook your leg around his side and bring him to you. This position gives you ample time for kissing. You can just take time to look into each other's eyes.

This position allows for wonderful stimulation of the clitoris while he gets the bonus of playing with your breasts and butt.

Glowing Juniper

Your man might need to be flexible for this position. He will sit down on the bed while you straddle him. Now lay down backward as your man lifts your hips and lower back and slowly slips in you. This position will give wonderful access to your G-spot while giving him the sensations of being deep inside you.

He has the advantage of playing with your breasts and clitoris. This position is more intense than just missionary or spooning, you will still feel closer since you are facing each other.

The Rock N Roller

This is a good position to get reacquainted with your partner since this is a great position to help you climax and he gets to see just how much you are enjoying what he is doing to you.

Get into the missionary position. After he has penetrated you, bring your legs up to rest on his chest or across his shoulders. He can support your rear with his hands or use them to explore your body.

He gets to be the dominant partner while you lay there being submissive. You can easily look into each other's eyes and kiss. Even though he is in the power position, you can set the pace together.

If you want to add some extra spark, wear heels and stockings.

The Amazon

Everybody loves having a prop handy when having sex. It doesn't get any hotter than have sex on a chair. Just imagine jumping into your partner's lap after a romantic home-cooked meal. You get extra points for raising up your skirt and keeping it on.

First, you need to get a chair and put your man in it. Now just climb on top and ease yourself onto his waiting member. Now just start grinding yourself against him while kissing him anyplace you can reach.

This position is great for orgasm as you are getting a lot of contact with your G-spot and clitoris. He is getting great sensations from being buried deep inside you.

The Lotus Blossom

The Lotus blossom is more natural and not as hard to get into. In this position, your man is going to sit in the lotus position. You will sit on him with your legs around his waist.

You will get the clitoral stimulation that you love and you can give him the speed and depth he wants. He is at your mercy in this position. Tell him to kiss your ears, neck, breasts, or anywhere he can reach.

The Sphinx

You might not like doggy style but will a few changes it can be very passionate. Doggy can be as romantic as any other position and it isn't just for animal sex.

Start off in normal doggy style but ask your partner to lean in closer over your back so he can kiss the back of your neck. You can also turn your head and capture his lips with yours.

Make sure you keep the close contact to make the doggy style more intimate. He is still in control but can kiss your back, neck, and mouth while bringing his hands up to play with your breasts.

The Side Kick

Just like the Sphinx, this position is about contact and is a true passionate position.

You will lie down on stomach with you head to one side. Your man will place one of his legs in between yours with the other one to the outside of your body. Your arms aren't of any use but his are free to wander where they want to.

He could massage your butt or back. He can grab your hair and pull gently to make him feel more in control.

Have him begin with long, slow thrusts and you will soon feel the true force of this position.

The Right Angle

You need a stable, hard surface like a kitchen counter or table. Now lie down on your back with your butt right on the edge. Your man will stand in between your legs and slowly enter you.

He has an amazing view of your body while the angle of penetration is great for your G-spot. It also makes you feel extra tight for him. What you do with your hands is totally up to you. Feel free to explore each other's bodies.

The Row Boat

Your man will lie down on his back. You are going to sit down on his hardened penis slowly. He will sit up and bring his knees and upper body up so that you are now face to face. His knees will be to the outside of your body. You will bend your knees and have them outside of his. You can also choose to wrap your legs around him.

Your man slips his arms over your calves and under your knees to your thighs so you can grip each other's hands. It looks kind of like the rocking position.

This position is intimate since you are face to face and looking into each other's eyes. You can also kiss each other for a more intimate bond. The penetration is slow and rocking. Try rocking together to create a thrusting motion.

Chapter 13: Alternative Sexual Experiences

For most people, threesomes, bondage, and anal sex only happen in movies. They don't have to be sequestered into the fantasy realm. With some planning, you can make your anal sex, bondage, or threesome a very sexual reality. Here is how.

Threesomes

If you have a partner that you are comfortable with, you need to pick your third partner carefully. It is a lot more complicated than staying away from best friends or ex-lovers. Relationship and sex experts say that finding one person in your friend group that you aren't that close to but is open to having a threesome. If you choose a stranger, you don't have to worry about long-term attachments, but you do risk not being attracted to the person you are getting ready to have sex with. There are also some safety hazards to take into consideration like sexually transmitted diseases.

If you are single, try dating sites that cater to people that are looking for multiple partners like POF. This also goes for Craigslist. Craigslist has a tendency to attract some weird people so you might want to FaceTime with them or meet them in person in a group setting first. There are some other sites like 3nder and FetLife that are interesting. You could always go to your local sex toy store and talk with people there. You could ask the people who work there or the owners what happens in the community and you might even find some fliers for other clubs or parties.

It doesn't matter if it is two women and a man or two men a one woman, it is totally up to you either as an individual or couple. Male-female-female is most common since guys are as open-minded about being with another man. With that said, women shouldn't cave just because her partner is forcing his preference on her.

If you haven't discussed this with your partner, you might need to suggest watching a movie about threesomes before outright asking your partner about having one. Once you see their reaction to the movie, you can ask them if they have had one or would be interested in having one.

If it goes well, you might casually ask them if they have anyone in mind to be their third. If you both agree to the person, then you need to approach them in a way, so you don't scare them off. Ask them casually like, "Hey, we think you are cool and fun. We would like to have a threesome, and we think we would have a lot of fun with you. Would you be interested?" If you already know the person, let them know that this will not change the friendship in any way. If it is someone you don't know, take time to get to know them first. Go out to dinner or drinks to see if you have a connection with them and feel like you can trust them.

Don't worry so much about asking. Most people on the receiving end will feel flattered.

You need to set some ground rules well in advance. You could think about taking sleepovers, oral sex, kissing, or possibly penetration off the table. Don't worry about taking activities off the table will make the experience worse, it could actually be more exciting without actually penetrating.

If you are in a relationship, you and your significant other could set up safe words or phrases you could use if things start to get too intense. Let the third person know they can speak up if they ever feel uncomfortable.

There are some things you need to have on hand. You are going to need plenty of condoms. If the man is penetrating each woman, he will need to take the condom off every time he changes partners. If he doesn't, he is exposing them to viruses, infections, and bacteria. Sex toys, lube, and toy cleaning wipes need to be on hand for wetness or added sensations. Toys need to be wiped down between partners, so you don't spread germs.

It is all easier said than done. Don't over-think things. Begin with a glass of wine and some appetizers. Start talking, and this will usually lead to flirting. Somebody will make a move in no time.

Massage is a good way to get intimate. There are massage candles that turn into an oil when blown out. This can be used to give a body rub that will set the mood.

The actual three-way needs to be organic. Maneuver, touch, and move any way you like. If you are a dominate person, take the lead. If not, let yourself be led and do what feels natural.

For some positions, the man could lay down on his back and receive oral sex from one partner while the other woman sits on his face and gets oral sex from him. A different position is one woman lies on her back while the other one lies on top of her. The guy penetrates the top woman doggy style, and the women can play with each other. Another option is to arrange everybody in a circle, and everyone performs oral sex on each other.

There is plenty of places to put mouths, genitals, and hands. If there is a free tongue or hand, find a place to put it.

Threesomes will take longer than normal sex, so you might need to change things up a lot. Guide your partners into ways you would like to do. Pay attention to any changes in the other's body language, sexual cues, and breathing patterns. Use movements to guide them, no words.

If it seems like someone is being left out, reach out and begin to play with them. This will help them to jump back in action.

You will need to figure out what you are going to do after the action beforehand. Let the others know. You might want just to say goodbye then, cuddle up for a while, or just hand out. Just remember to talk about what is expected of everyone, so no one is surprised later on. If a sleepover is planned, the third party needs to know in advance so they can pack an overnight bag.

Bondage

If bondage is new to you and your partner, bring up the subject gently, so they won't freak out. During sex, begin by pinning your partner's hands down and telling them that they are now at your mercy. Let this be a starting point to the conversation about pushing the subject of bondage more.

Blindfolds are a great place to start since they don't feel as strange as handcuffs might. Not being able to see will help some get rid of their inhibitions. Take turns blindfolding the other and then treat them to sensations like, kissing, tickling, lightly scratching, and licking your partner in various places, so they don't have a clue as to what is going to happen next. This will mirror the sensations that happen when tying up your partner.

Before you bring out the handcuffs and ropes, you must choose a safe word if things start getting too intense for the submissive. Try the word yellow if you want the dominant one to ease up but not stop. The word red shows your partner that you want to stop completely. The safe word should never be stop or no since saying these things gives the dominant the right to override your protests. Getting your demands overridden is part of the fun of being out of control.

You should only try bondage with someone you feel 100 percent safe with. Now, set a timer for 30 minutes for your first session because it will be extremely intense. Don't use gags or blindfolds for the first few times. Just try tying up the submissive partner, so you learn to read each other. Do not ever leave a person that is tied up alone.

If you think you are ready to push the envelope, start by using a soft rope or silk scarves to tie up your submissive partner up with in different ways. Allow the dominant to configure the rope into a figure eight that goes between the breasts and behind your back. This will push up your breasts and accentuate them. A different scenario has them stand with their arms at their sides and wrap the rope around the torso, so their arms are tied down. Just be creative, let the rope twist over their body any way that feels right. Touch them sexually with your fingers as you pull the rope across and through their body parts. When you finally have them tied up challenge them to escape. Stay away from the neck area. If you decide to tie their ankles together, be sure they can't fall. Never, ever use bungee cords, these will snap and hurt your partner. Don't tie them up too tight. You should be able to slip a finger between the rope and their body. They shouldn't feel any numbness or pain.

The handcuffs you decide to will help to set the tone. Metal or leather will make you feel like a bad ass where a fuzzy pair will have you feeling playful. Begin by binding your partner's hands together either in front or behind their backs. Move on to a position where they are secured to the bed with their arms up and out to the sides. Never use cheap costume handcuffs. These can tighten and hurt your partner. Don't use stocking as these can cut into the skin.

The dominant partner needs to move into things by starting out sensual and sweet. Think about kissing softly and slowly. It is extremely hot being tied up but yet being treated very tenderly. As the game progresses, the dominant one can bring out their inner tiger.

For another naughty twist, wrap up certain body parts in plastic wrap, like around your hips and breasts. This plastic drives him wild since he will be able to see but not touch you. When you have him good and worked up, allow him to have his way. Have some blunt tipped scissors near so they can cut you lose.

Another hot idea is to tie your partner up with toilet paper. Be sure to twist it to make it stronger. Tell them they can't break free and then tantalize them until they can't stand it. When they rip loose, then you can punish them.

If you want to take it up a notch, try using a spreader bar. It will hold your partner's legs apart so you can have your way with them.

Role-playing can help transition into bondage. A few fun games are: pirate/princess, prison guard/prisoner, cop/robber, burglar/defenseless housewife.

The biggest part of what makes bondage so pleasurable is the aspect of not allowing your partner to have pleasure. If they are tied up, begin by slowly stripping in front of them. Let them watch as you touch yourself. When they are begging you to touch them, begin by slowly stroking their most intimate parts and then penetrate them slowly. Tell them that they can't have an orgasm until you tell them to.

If both partners agree to be both dominant and submissive, switch between these roles, and you will be amazed at what will get you going.

Anal

Of all the numerous sex acts, Anal remains the most misunderstood. Anal sex is not the first thing when you think about mutually pleasurable things you want to do with your partner. The urban legend states that "Guys want it since they think it is tighter than a vagina. They have seen it in porn, and women use it as a bargaining chip for special occasions."

Quite frankly, that is pure crap. A lot of women do it just because they like it.

The main thing other women want to know is will it hurt?

All women will agree that yes, it does hurt the first few times. The main thing to remember is to relax. Don't think about it. Prepare for it. It won't be as bad if you begin with lube and fingers. Widening the hole before penetration can help it not hurt as bad.

Why do you want to do it?

Mostly because it is considered to be taboo and naughty. Some do it to impress the guy they are with after a night of partying. Having anal sex when you are extremely turned on is more pleasurable. Some women can have an orgasm during anal sex. The ones who do orgasm during anal, say it is more intense than a normal orgasm.

Who wants it more, the woman or man?

Most women say that their men were the one who initiated anal sex. Most women concede due to the fact they don't want to hurt their men's feelings. They don't want their man to think they aren't into them. Some have been lucky, and it was mutually wanted. Most men are infatuated with anal sex and butts.

How does it feel the first time?

It is very weird. It is very tight and unpleasant. It is a bad cramp. Just like you are stretching a muscle that has never been used before. If you can make yourself relax and be prepared, it will be better.

What will it feel like after you have done it for a while?

It makes you feel like you are completely full. Very intense. You learn to adjust just like you did with normal sex. With time, you know what you are going to fill and learn to enjoy it. It won't hurt as bad since you aren't as nervous. The initial penetration will always feel weird, but once you get going, it is enjoyable.

Will it ever feel good?

If the person you are with lets you control the force and speed; it can be quite pleasurable. It also depends on the size of the man's penis. If you can combine it with clitoral and vaginal stimulation, it can feel great.

Is waxing a necessity?

No, most decent guys don't care what a female looks like back there. If you feel more comfortable, then, by all means, go for it.

How soon into a relationship should it happen?

If the guy has a fetish for this sort of thing, it is really hard to hide, and he will bring it up right away. Most will wait six months or more until you have thoroughly enjoyed each other in all other intimate ways.

To lube or not to lube?

If you don't want it to hurt and feel horrible, lots of lube is needed. They type is up to you. Use whatever you have on hand or your favorite. If you find yourself out of lube but have coconut oil on hand, that works just as well.

Will you bleed?

You shouldn't bleed as long as the guy takes precautions and uses lube. If he forces himself into you, it is possible.

Do you need to protect the bed with towels?

Anal sex isn't messier than normal sex. If you are a squirter, or just get extremely wet during sex, then use a towel.

What is the cleanup like?

There isn't any cleanup. Just the normal lube and wetness. The condom is the only thing that needs to be taken off.

Are there certain positions or angles to try?

Most say the doggy style is the easiest and most convenient. Some women find it pleasurable with the girl on top so she can control the pace.

Are condoms still required?

Absolutely, condoms are still and will always be a requirement.

Can you have an orgasm from anal sex alone?

Usually not. If you can stimulate the clitoris along with anal sex, you will probably have an orgasm. Don't worry about it if you can't. It is all about what you feel with your partner and how they make you feel. Just enjoy yourself and have fun.

Conclusion

Thank for making it through to the end of *Sex Guide for Women*. Let's hope it was informative and able to provide you with all of the tools you need to achieve your goals of achieving the sexual desire of your dreams.

The next step is to put the information in this book to good use. Start trying some of these tips. Decide what area you need to work on the most and start to make some changes. You deserve to open up your sexual desire, so get started today.

DEAR reader,

Thank you for reading to end of this 3-in-1 bundle. We hope you liked the book and the bundle format!

If you want more of these bundles, please check out our other books in the Sex Life Bundle Series!